Neurogenic Communication Disorders and the Life Participation Approach

THE SOCIAL IMPERATIVE IN SUPPORTING INDIVIDUALS AND FAMILIES

Neurogenic Communication Disorders and the Life Participation Approach

THE SOCIAL IMPERATIVE IN SUPPORTING INDIVIDUALS AND FAMILIES

Audrey L. Holland
PhD, CCC-SLP, BC-ANCDS
Roberta J. Elman
PhD, CCC-SLP, BC-ANCDS

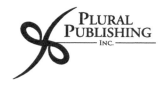

PLURAL PUBLISHING INC.

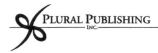
PLURAL PUBLISHING
INC.

5521 Ruffin Road
San Diego, CA 92123

e-mail: information@pluralpublishing.com
Website: https://www.pluralpublishing.com

Typeset in 11/13 Garamond by Flanagan's Publishing Services, Inc.
Printed in the United States of America by Integrated Books International
23 22 21 20   2 3 4 5

Library of Congress Cataloging-in-Publication Data

Names: Holland, Audrey L., editor. | Elman, Roberta J., editor.
Title: Neurogenic communication disorders and the life participation
   approach : the social imperative in supporting individuals and families
   / [edited by] Audrey L. Holland, Roberta J. Elman.
Description: San Diego, CA : Plural Publishing, [2021] | Includes
   bibliographical references and index.
Identifiers: LCCN 2020016177 | ISBN 9781635502954 (paperback) | ISBN
   1635502950 (paperback) | ISBN 9781635502893 (ebook)
Subjects: MESH: Aphasia—therapy | Communication Disorders—therapy |
   Patient Participation | Patient-Centered Care | Life Style | Quality of
   Life
Classification: LCC RC425 | NLM WL 340.5 | DDC 616.85/52—dc23
LC record available at https://lccn.loc.gov/2020016177

CONTENTS

PREFACE

$\mathcal{W}$hen Amy Hanson from SpeechPathology.com asked me to organize a symposium on Life Participation in Aphasia for their online educational service, I jumped at the chance. The symposium was to be conducted for one week, one hour a day for five weekdays. And I knew immediately what I wanted to do: capture one writer of the LPAA statement, and surround her with four "youngsters" to the 20+ year-old movement. Roberta Elman was my first choice, and she said yes. I then gathered a list of possible others, which was considerable, and rather arbitrarily chose four who had different interests, to join Roberta. I wanted relative newbies, because I thought it was time for new voices to be heard, but I had scads of backups. (The world is changing!!) AND all four said yes! I, who am a visual rather than auditory learner, planned to listen to all the webinars, of course, but with pain. Surprise! When Friday rolled around and it was over, I had learned, and enjoyed every single minute of the listening. Thinking to strike while the iron was still hot, I called each participant and asked (Roberta first) if they would be interested in turning the whole thing into a book. Once again, all said yes! And I decided to reach into my bag of tricks and find a few more. Once again, original speakers were joined by two more first choices, and we were off and running. You will note that some of the co-authors might have more familiar names. First authors chose them, as they saw fit. Others went with less familiar people. Finally, we felt flattered when Nina Simmons-Mackie agreed to take a last look over everyone's efforts. So what we have here are essentially young voices, joined in some cases by other young voices, or by more experienced ones. We hope you enjoy, but more importantly LEARN from reading our efforts about the history of the movement, some treatment and assessment approaches that can fit into the strictures of current day health care, and provide ideas for moving away from simply concentrating on the impairments but moving on to how whose impairments have impact on everyday life.

—ALH

When Audrey Holland asked me to be part of the webinar series, I was truly honored and excited! Being part of a project that focused on helping clinicians apply a life participation approach to their own practice had become part of my life's mission. And my excitement rose higher when Audrey shared the idea of creating a book based on the five webinars, plus adding contributions from a few others. The current book represents our collective efforts.

In the prologue to the book, you will find the Life Participation Approach to Aphasia (LPAA) article that was originally published in the *ASHA Leader* in 2000. This serves as a foundation for the nine chapters that follow. First up is Audrey's chapter. In it, she weaves her personal career together with the "life participation movement" and its leaders throughout the English-speaking world. In Chapter 2, I share the ups and downs of my own career trajectory toward implementing LPAA, ending with development of the C.A.P.E. checklist. Sarah Baar, in Chapter 3, shares her tips, tricks, and tools for bringing LPAA into your own clinical practice. In Chapter 4, Tom Sather and Tami Howe focus on the important role of the environment in supporting language, communication, and participation, especially for individuals who are living with aphasia. Katie Strong and Barbara Shadden, in Chapter 5, reveal the benefits of helping clients to share their own personal narratives, in order to support identity. In Chapter 6, Becky Khayum and Aimee Mooney provide clinicians with a roadmap for incorporating person-centered intervention, especially for clients who are living with primary progressive aphasia. Natalie Douglas and Delainey Smyth, in Chapter 7, show clinicians how they can apply a life participation intervention approach for people living with dementia. In Chapter 8, Peter Meulenbroek and Louise Keegan, share how to apply a life participation focus for those with traumatic brain injury. And, finally, in Chapter 9, Nina Simmons-Mackie completes the book with her thoughts on the past, present, and future of LPAA.

—*RJE*

We hope you find this book inspiring and relevant to your present or future clinical practice!

ACKNOWLEDGMENTS

Audrey: In remembrance of four visionaries: Mike Adler, Pat Arato, Shirley Morgenstein, and Claire Penn.

Roberta: To the people and creatures who have enriched my life participation . . .

CONTRIBUTORS

Sarah Baar, MA, CCC-SLP
Honeycomb Speech Therapy
Ada, Michigan
Chapter 3

Natalie F. Douglas, PhD, CCC-SLP
Associate Professor
Central Michigan University
Mount Pleasant, Michigan
Chapter 7

Roberta J. Elman, PhD, CCC-SLP, BC-ANCDS
President and Founder
Aphasia Center of California
Oakland and Menlo Park, California
Chapter 2

Audrey L. Holland, PhD, CCC-SLP, BC-ANCDS
Regents' Professor Emerita
University of Arizona
Department of Speech, Language, and Hearing Sciences
University of Arizona
Tucson, Arizona
Chapter 1

Tami J. Howe, PhD
Assistant Professor
School of Audiology and Speech Sciences
Faculty of Medicine
University of British Colombia
Vancouver, British Colombia, Canada
Chapter 4

Louise C. Keegan, PhD, CCC-SLP
Associate Professor
Program Director of Speech-Language Pathology
Moravian College
Bethlehem, Pennsylvania
Chapter 8

Rebecca Khayum, MS, CCC-SLP
President, Memory Care Corporation
Adjunct Instructor
Northwestern Mesulam Center for Cognitive Neurology and
    Alzheimer's Disease
Chicago, Illinois
Chapter 6

Peter Meulenbroek, PhD, CCC-SLP
Assistant Professor
Department of Communication Sciences and Disorders
Director
Social Communication and Cognitive Abilities Lab
Lexington, Kentucky
Chapter 8

Aimee R. Mooney, MS, CCC-SLP
Assistant Professor
Oregon Health and Science University
Institute on Development and Disability
Assistant Clinical Professor
Portland State University
Speech and Hearing Sciences Department
Portland, Oregon
Chapter 6

Thomas W. Sather, PhD, CCC-SLP
Associate Professor
Communication Sciences and Disorders
University of Wisconsin-Eau Claire
Speech-Language Pathologist
Department of Rehabilitation Services
Mayo Clinic Health System

Eau Claire, Wisconsin
Chapter 4

Barbara B. Shadden, PhD, CCC-SLP, BC-ANCDS
University Professor Emerita
Program in Communication Disorders
University of Arkansas
Fayetteville, Arkansas
Chapter 5

Nina Simmons-Mackie, PhD
Professor Emeritus
Southeastern Louisiana University
Hammond, Louisiana
Chapter 9

Delainey Smyth, BA
Graduate Student
Central Michigan University
Mount Pleasant, Michigan
Chapter 7

Katie A. Strong, PhD, CCC-SLP
Assistant Professor
Department of Communication Sciences and Disorders
Central Michigan University
Mount Pleasant, Michigan
Chapter 5

PROLOGUE
Life Participation Approach to Aphasia: A Statement of Values for the Future*

LPAA Project Group

(in alphabetical order): *Roberta Chapey, Judith F. Duchan, Roberta J. Elman, Linda J. Garcia, Aura Kagan, Jon G. Lyon, and Nina Simmons-Mackie*

$\mathcal{U}$nprecedented changes are occurring in the way treatment for aphasia is viewed—and reimbursed. These changes, resulting from both internal and external pressures, are influencing how speech-language pathologists carry out their jobs.

Internal influences include a growing interest in treatments that produce meaningful real life outcomes leading to enhanced quality of life. Externally, we are influenced by disability rights activists encouraging adjustments in philosophy and treatment, and by consumers frustrated by unmet needs and unfulfilled goals. Most recently, a strong external influence is emanating from the curtailment of funding for our work that has caused a significant reduction in available services to people affected by aphasia.

To accommodate these varied influences on service delivery, it is important to take a proactive stance. We therefore propose a philosophy of service delivery that meets the needs of people affected by aphasia and confronts the pressures from our profession, providers, and funding sources.

Our statement of values has been guided by the ideas and work of speech-language pathologists as well as by individuals in psychology, sociology, and medicine. We intend neither to prescribe exact methods for achieving specific outcomes, nor

*Originally published as: LPAA Project Group (In alphabetical order: Roberta Chapey, Judith F. Duchan, Roberta J. Elman, Linda J. Garcia, Aura Kagan, Jon G. Lyon, & Nina Simmons Mackie) (2000). *ASHA Leader, 5*(3), 4–6 https://doi.org/10.1044/leader.FTR.05032000.4. Reprinted with permission from the American Speech-Language-Hearing Association.

to provide a quick fix to the challenges facing our profession. Rather, we offer a statement of values and ideas relevant to assessment, intervention, policy making, advocacy, and research that we hope will stimulate discussion related to restructuring of services and lead to innovative clinical methods for supporting those affected by aphasia.

Defining the Approach

The "Life Participation Approach to Aphasia" (LPAA) is a consumer-driven service-delivery approach that supports individuals with aphasia and others affected by it in achieving their immediate and longer term life goals (note that "approach" refers here to a general philosophy and model of service delivery, rather than to a specific clinical approach). LPAA calls for a broadening and refocusing of clinical practice and research on the consequences of aphasia. It focuses on re-engagement in life, beginning with initial assessment and intervention, and continuing, after hospital discharge, until the consumer no longer elects to have communication support.

LPAA places the life concerns of those affected by aphasia at the center of all decision making It empowers the consumer to select and participate in the recovery process and to collaborate on the design of interventions that aim for a more rapid return to active life. These interventions thus have the potential to reduce the consequences of disease and injury that contribute to long-term health costs.

The Essence of LPAA

We encourage clinicians and researchers to focus on the real-life goals of people affected by aphasia. For example, in the initial stages following a CVA, a goal may be to establish effective communication with the surrounding nursing staff and physicians. At a later stage, a life goal may be to return to employment or participation in the local community.

Regardless of the stage of management, LPAA emphasizes the attainment of re-engagement in life by strengthening daily participation in activities of choice. Residual skill is thus seen as only one of many requisites. For example, full participation is dependent on motivation and a consistent and dependable support system. A highly supportive environment can lessen the consequences of aphasia on one's life, whatever the language impairment. A nonsupportive environment, on the other hand, can substantially increase the chance of aphasia affecting daily routines. Someone with mild aphasia in a nonsupportive environment might experience greater daily encumbrances than another with severe aphasia who is highly supported.

In this broadening and refocusing of services, LPAA recommends that clinicians and researchers consider the dual function of communication—transmitting and receiving messages and establishing and maintaining social links. Furthermore, life activities do not need to be in the realm of communication in order to deserve or receive intervention. What is important is to judge whether aphasia affects the execution of activities of choice and one's involvement in them (see Table 0–1 for a few examples of how LPAA may lead to a broadening and refocusing of services).

The Origins of LPAA

Functional and Pragmatic Approaches

LPAA draws on ideas underlying functional and pragmatic approaches to aphasia and shares some common values with those who take a broad approach to functional communication treatment by focusing on life participation goals and social relationships. In our view, however, the term "functional" does not do justice to the breadth of this work. In addition, the term is often used narrowly to mean "functional independence in getting a message across." Although LPAA recognizes the value of this type of impairment-level work, it should form part of a bigger picture where the ultimate goal for intervention is re-engagement into everyday society.

Table 0–1. Examples of the Shift in Focus of Life Participation Approach to Aphasia

LPAA	Examples of Shift in Focus
Assessment includes determining relevant life participation needs and discovering clients' competencies.	In addition to assessing language and communication deficits, clinicians are equally interested in assessing how the person with aphasia does with support.
Treatment includes facilitating the achievement of life goals.	In addition to work on improving and/or compensating for the language impairment, clinicians are prepared to work on anything in which aphasia is a barrier to life participation (even if the activity is not directly related to communication).
Intervention routinely targets environmental factors outside of the individual.	In addition to working with the individual on language or compensatory functional-communication techniques, clinicians might train communication partners, or work on other ways of reducing barriers to make the environment more "aphasia-friendly."
All those affected by aphasia are regarded as legitimate targets for intervention.	In addition to working with the individual who has aphasia, clinicians would also work on life participation goals for family and others who are affected by the aphasia, including friends, service providers, work colleagues, etc.
Clinician roles are expanded beyond those of teacher or therapist.	In addition to doing therapy, clinicians might take on the role of: • "communication partner," and give the person with aphasia the opportunity to engage in conversation about life goals, concerns about the future, barriers to life participation, etc. • "coach," "problem solver," or "support person" in relation to overcoming challenges in reengaging in a particular life activity
Outcome evaluation involves routinely documenting quality of life and life participation changes.	In addition to documenting changes in language and communication, clinicians would routinely evaluate the following in partnership with clients: • life activities and how satisfying they are, • social connections and how satisfying they are, • emotional well-being.

Human Rights Issues and Consumers' Goals

LPAA is a means of addressing unmet needs and rights of individuals with aphasia and those in their environment. Indeed, the Americans with Disabilities Act (ADA), signed into law on July 26, 1990, requires that physical and communication access be provided for individuals with aphasia and other disabilities and allows them legal recourse if they are blocked from accessing employment, programs, and services in the public and private sectors.

In 1992, ASHA provided guidelines for a "communication bill of rights" (National Joint Committee for the Communicative Needs of Persons with Severe Disabilities). Its preface states that "all persons, regardless of the extent or severity of their disabilities, have a basic right to affect, through communication, the conditions of their own existence." Communication is defined as "a basic need and basic right of all human beings" (p. 2). ASHA thus views communication as an integral part of life participation.

Emphasis on Competence and Inclusion

LPAA philosophy embraces a view of treatment that emphasizes competence and inclusion in daily life, focusing as much on the consequences of chronic disorders as on the language difficulty caused by the aphasia. Along with other movements in education and health care, LPAA shifts from a focus on deficits and remediation to one of inclusion and life participation (see Fougeyrollas et al., 1997; WHO, ICIDH-2, 1997). Such international changes in focus point to the need to address the personal experience of disability and promote optimal life inclusion and reintegration into society.

Changes in Reimbursement and Service Delivery

Health care and reimbursement in America have undergone an unprecedented overhaul. Financial exigencies have led to an emphasis on medically essential treatments and others seen as likely to save on future health care costs. Many of the incentives in this model result in the provision of efficient short-term minimal care, rather than the longer term, fuller care supported in the past.

LPAA represents a fundamental shift in how we view service delivery for people confronting aphasia. Since LPAA focuses on broader life-related processes and outcomes from the onset of treatment, service delivery and its reimbursement will require novel means that stand outside most current practices. We are confident that cost-sensitive and therapeutically effective models are possible. Our purpose in this introductory article is to prompt a discussion with providers and consumers as to whether life participation principles and values should play a more central role in the delivery and reimbursement of future service delivery for all those affected by aphasia.

The Core Values of LPAA

LPAA is structured around five core values that serve as guides to assessment, intervention, and research.

The Explicit Goal Is Enhancement of Life Participation

In the LPAA approach, the first focus of the client, clinician, and policy-maker is to assess the extent to which persons affected by aphasia are able to achieve life participation goals, and the extent to which the aphasia hinders the attainment of these desired outcomes. The second focus is to improve short- and long-term participation in life.

Everyone Affected by Aphasia Is Entitled to Service

LPAA supports all those affected directly by aphasia, including immediate family and close associates of the adult with aphasia. The LPAA approach holds that it is essential to build protected communities within society where persons with aphasia are able not only to participate but are valued as participants. Therefore, intervention may involve changing broader social systems to make them more accessible to those affected by aphasia.

Success Measures Include Documented Life-Enhancement Changes

The LPAA approach calls for the use of outcome measures that assess quality of life and the degree to which those affected by aphasia meet their life participation goals.

Without a cause to communicate, we believe there is no practical need for communication. Therefore, treatment focuses on a reason to communicate as much as on communication repair. In so doing, treatment attends to each consumer's feelings, relationships, and activities in life.

Both Personal and Environmental Factors Are Intervention Targets

Disruption of daily life for individuals affected by aphasia (including those who do not have aphasia themselves) is evident on two levels: personal (internal) and environmental (external). Intervention consists of constantly assessing, weighing, and prioritizing which personal and environmental factors should be targets of intervention and how best to provide freer, easier, and more autonomous access to activities and social connections of choice. This does not mean that treatment comprises only life resumption processes, but rather that enhanced participation in life "governs" management from its inception. In this fundamental way, the LPAA approach differs from one in which life enhancement is targeted only after language repair has been addressed.

Emphasis Is on the Availability of Services as Needed at All Stages of Aphasia

LPAA begins with the onset of aphasia and continues until consumers and providers agree that targeted life enhancement changes have occurred. However, LPAA acknowledges that life consequences of aphasia change over time and should be addressed regardless of the length of time post-onset. Consumers are therefore permitted to discontinue intervention, and reenter treatment when they believe they need to continue work on a goal or to attain a new life goal.

Conclusions

Our health-care systems are undergoing change and, as a result, so are our professions. How we allow this change to affect our clinical practice, our research directions, and our response to consumer advocacy is up to us. We need to educate policy-makers that being fiscally responsible means having a consumer-driven model of intervention focusing on interventions that make real-life differences and minimize the consequences of disease and injury.

While it is clear that the implicit motivation underlying all clinical and research efforts in aphasia is related to increased participation in life, the path to achieving that goal is often indirect. Because LPAA makes life goals primary and explicit, it holds promise as an approach in which such goals are attainable. We invite other speech-language pathologists to join us in discussing and developing life participation approaches to aphasia.

Short List of References Published with the Original Article

Fougeyrollas, P., Cloutier, R., Bergeron, H., Cote, J., Cote, M., & St. Michel, G. (1997). *Revision of the Quebec Classification: Handicap creation process.* Lac St-Charles, Quebec: International Network on the Handicap Creation Process.

National Joint Committee for the Communicative Needs of Persons with Severe Disabilities. (1992). Guidelines for meeting the communication needs of persons with severe disabilities. *ASHA, 34* (March, Suppl. 7), 1–8.

World Health Organization. (1997). *International classification of impairments, activities and participation: A manual of dimensions of disablement and functions. Beta-1 draft for field trials.* Geneva, Switzerland: WHO.

For the detailed list of references published with the original article, please go to the Aphasia Institute's website: http://www .aphasia.ca

THE SOCIAL IMPERATIVE FOR APHASIA REHABILITATION

A PERSONAL HISTORY

Audrey L. Holland

Aphasia is not life threatening, but it stops people from having a life.

—Pat Arato, "The Language Thief"

Background

Roberta and I deliberately chose younger clinicians and researchers to write chapters in this book, although they were free to choose the "older guard" as coauthors. We believe that fresh new approaches are badly needed so that the "Social Imperative" can continue to grow and be productive. My task was to share its 50-year-old history as I have seen it develop to this point.

Isn't the Social Imperative what good therapy is all about? Well, yes and no. I believe that test score changes and more focused pre-post changes as a result of specific, language-focused training regimens, are of equal value. Understanding the impairments and learning to use the specific techniques that improve core language impairments are vitally important. We know that for aphasia and TBI, improvement is likely to occur as a function of appropriate, impairment-focused treatment. However, it is not enough. For individuals with dementia and PPA, the scenario is different. Here, the goal is to help people maintain their language skills for as long as possible.

There is another problem as well. The current health care system fails to recognize that all of these disorders are chronic. Only limited benefits extend beyond the earliest periods of actually living with the disorder. This, then, is part of the Social Imperative. Under the current circumstances, how can the lingering consequences be minimized most efficiently and effectively? It is extremely important for prospective clinicians that their curricula be rearranged so that they can learn about these concerns and newer, impairment-focused intervention skills that address them.

A Brief, Clinically-Focused History of Aphasia Study

The elusive and exotic language disorder called aphasia that frequently accompanies brain injury or other neurologic conditions has intrigued physicians, philosophers, and scientists since 3500 BC (Benton & Joint, 1960). Their interest was (and still seems to be) how aphasia could inform questions of the neuroanatomical localization of language, as well as furthering our understanding of human beings' unique ability to have developed and use it.

Concern with what could be done to rehabilitate language, although sporadic before the end of World War I, became intense in Germany and Russia as the war ended, and as young, head-injured men struggled to live normal lives despite their difficulties in speaking and talking. The United States and most of the English-speaking world, however, showed only limited interest before the conclusion of World War II.[1] The increased interest was due to the influx of substantial numbers of head-injured veterans coming home after that war. In the United States, hospitals and training programs were developed at military and then Veteran's Administration hospitals across the country. The pioneers in this effort included Hildred Schuell, Ollie Backus, Jon Eisenson, and Kurt Goldstein (bringing his European knowledge) among many others.

Foremost among these was Joseph Wepman, who directed the program at DeWitt General Hospital in California. Dr. Wepman's *Recovery from Aphasia* (1951) became my Sirius, my guide star. But it was all fairly abstract for me, because I did not even know anybody with aphasia until after I obtained my doctorate. I was just intrigued by the problem.

My personal history in aphasia started in the early 1960s, when l took my first academic job at Emerson College in Boston, also the location of the renowned Boston VA Hospital. I managed to talk my way into attending the Aphasia Grand Rounds there, conducted by Norman Geschwind, Harold Goodglass, Edith Kaplan, and Robert Sparks, who all took pity on me and became my mentors. I finally met my first person with aphasia there.

At that time, I was a flaming behaviorist, planning to remedy aphasia with carefully chosen language stimuli based on frequencies of occurrence and such abstract notions, flawlessly appropriate schedules of reinforcement, and well-developed techniques for shaping behavior and such. The VA was a spectacular place to see creative personal, impairment-focused work in assessment and treatment as it was conducted by Sparks, Goodglass, Kaplan, and a bit later, by Nancy Helm-Estabrooks. Nevertheless, I persisted (so to speak). I held fast to my behaviorist principles and planned to adapt all of the wonderful things I was learning into Skinnerian terms.

But being in the rich intellectual world of Boston and Cambridge, I found myself intrigued with other thoughts, of my own

---

[1]A very concise history of aphasia can be found on the internet by searching for "History of Aphasia."

thoughts, such as: If aphasia is a language disorder, a language is used to communicate, to fully relive life, and to get along with others, then aphasia must surely affect the larger world of communication, not just its language part!

This was the heyday for people who were interested in what was coming to be known as language pragmatics. This was nuanced, perhaps, but clearly a more real world of speakers and listeners collaborating to exchange messages. This was the world of Grice (1975) with his timeless Cooperative Principles for how speakers and listeners interact to create verbal interaction; of Austin, (whose influence was well known then but his earlier Harvard essays were not published until 1975); and Searle's (1969) incisive analysis, "Speech Acts," that is, that meaning results from interaction between speakers and listener. I thought it was extremely important to try to connect language pragmatics to aphasia rehabilitation. I pondered what is still one of my favorite rationales, that of Watzlawick, Beavin, and Jackson (1967) to the effect that "Humans cannot not communicate." So, I read a lot, and strived to attend a lot of the endless number of lectures that contributed so much to the Boston-Cambridge intellectual reputation.

AND I finally began to work with my first aphasic client. MS was a young graduate student when he incurred aphasia as a result of an arteriovenous malformation (AVM) bleed. He was bright, eager, and optimistic about working hard to bring about his (substantial) recovery. We slogged through a whole lot of behavioral training, and MS certainly improved. But somehow, my role seemed more related to my counseling background than to my stimulus-response skills. I was far more interested in how his changed career plans, his negotiations through life, and his marriage were influenced by his aphasia. I just didn't know what to do about any of it, except to listen and to counsel, and make tentative suggestions for him to try out. I don't quite know how I helped, but, he survived me. MS went on to become a successful marriage counselor with a solid clinical reputation. And at least my "treatment" caused no long-term harm.

And that is how I began to discover who I think I am today. I probably would have gotten here sooner or later, but it would have taken much longer if I had not encountered the Boston Veterans Administration Hospital, language pragmatics, communication, and finally, the work of Martha Taylor Sarno.

Martha Taylor Sarno and the Functional Communication Profile (FCP) (1969)

Sarno's inventory, the FCP, was published at the end of that decade. This was a big step away from available tests of language impairment and loss. It made perfect sense to me: asking systematic questions about how someone was getting along after aphasia has entered their everyday lives and finding out about the areas that were working well despite aphasia . . . or not. THIS is what was aphasia rehabilitation should be about.

Martha Taylor Sarno is the Founding Mother of the Social Imperative. She initiated the Social Imperative by exploring how persons with aphasia (PWA) and their spouses go about getting on with life, not necessarily what the "experts" might have to tell them about language processing and word retrieval. Sarno had to have recognized the Social Imperative before 1969, of course. However, it seems safe to assume that her priceless contribution to "functional communication" in the fullest sense of the word, began in 1969, and essentially has never stopped. It is important to note that Martha Sarno went on to form the National Aphasia Association (NAA). Its reins were handed over to the multi-talented Darlene Williamson in 2012, and since then, the NAA has continued to grow, thrive, and make significant contributions to living well with aphasia. It is also true that Sarno was a founding member of the impairment-research oriented Academy of Aphasia, a group she (nor I) never abandoned. I feel comfortable in her and my shared beliefs that both the impairment of aphasia and its consequences require our research and clinical attention.

This is being written in 2019, which is the Golden Anniversary of the Social Imperative in American Aphasiology. The FCP has since been joined by what seem to me to be hundreds of inventories looking at hundreds of aspects of social communication in aphasia and other language disorders, tons of ways to measure and to treat it. Nevertheless, it started with the FCP inventory.

The 1960s also figured prominently in the early history of the Social Imperative in a therapeutic way. In 1965, the American actress, Patricia Neal, suffered a life-threatening and aphasia-producing cerebral aneurysm. Her return to health and the resumption of her storied career were in large measure orchestrated by her husband, Roald Dahl, the prolific writer of children's books. Dahl planned her post-hospital treatments himself. His unique approach had profound influence, ultimately, on the Social Imperative. Dahl had friends and family come to their home and interact with Ms. Neal for an hour each day, for a total of six hours of talk and social interaction in an effort to help his wife speak again.

This approach was subsequently used successfully by Pat Arato in Toronto in the rehabilitation of her ex-husband, Oscar. Arato then extended this work to a small group of persons with aphasia and some volunteers. According to Kagan and Gailey (1993), Pat Arato's goal was "to give people hope; to help them to talk; to let them know that their life had not come to an end and there was somewhere for them to go." Her "small group" ultimately became the Pat Arato Center in suburban Toronto, founded in 1979. This center, now the famed Aphasia Institute, was the first in North America. The institute has had worldwide influence on the Social Imperative.

The Seventies and Eighties

Child language work introduced pragmatics and social concerns into speech-language pathology in the 1970s. This was largely through the groundbreaking research and scholarship of Elizabeth Bates. Bates gave our field a philosophical and linguistic gift in 1976, with her book *Language in Context: The Acquisition of Pragmatics;* and in all of her work that followed until the too early end of her life in 2003. Bates' interest at first was in child language, but it later grew to include aphasia as well (Dick et al., 2001). She left an indelible mark upon our history.

Liz Bates was a valued and important friend and colleague. Her influence on me was both direct and indirect. I don't remember the circumstances of our first meeting, but I DO remember the instant connection. Liz later introduced me to her friend and co-author, Brian MacWhinney when he joined the faculty at Carnegie Mellon University in Pittsburgh. (By 1970, I had moved to Pittsburgh and my alma mater, the University of Pittsburgh.)

Some years later, that friendship resulted in our collaboration on the development of AphasiaBank, the repository of aphasic language (comprehensively described most recently by Fromm, Forbes, Holland, & MacWhinney, 2020). In 1975, I was awarded a federal contract to develop a measure of functional communication. The result was the test, Communicative Activities of Daily Living (CADL), developed in 1980, and now in its 3rd edition (Holland, 2018). The CADL is grounded in "speech acts," as defined by Searle, noted earlier and remains so through two subsequent editions. But for me, the broader world of life participation opened up with CADL as well. The groundwork of the 1970s affected clinical workers across the Western world, of course, but being a practicing monolinguist, my work has centered mostly on clinicians and clinical researchers in the English-speaking world. Thus, this chapter reflects my own narrowed worldview of aphasia. In the 1980s, the field burgeoned, and new figures were emerging.

My first entrance into this larger world occurred when I was invited to South Africa in the early 1980s. There, I met the late Claire Penn, who had been a post-doctoral student of Carol Prutting. Claire influenced my personal and professional life until she died in 2018. She carried her lifelong interests and research in language pragmatics across the spectrum, from congenital deafness to aphasia. Ultimately, she influenced the even broader area of health communication in South Africa, where her legacy will continue to be felt for many years to come. However, it was her early work in aphasia and language pragmatics that remains central to the concerns of this chapter. See Penn (1993) for an elegant synthesis of it.

I also met Aura Kagan in South Africa before she immigrated to Canada. Her influence on me was similarly deep. Both Claire and Aura came from more traditional training: in linguistics, for Claire in Great Britain, and for Aura in psychology at the University of Witwatersrand, South Africa. Both felt that their earlier backgrounds helped, but did not quite mesh with the interpersonal and social needs that they believed were common among people with aphasia. They both sought to combine their more traditional training with the richer fields of sociolinguistics, pragmatics, and so forth. More about Aura Kagan later in this chapter.

And then, there were the United Kingdom and Australia. The Social Imperative was immeasurably influenced by Britons, like Sally Byng and Carole Pound, their germinal program at Aphasia Connect in London, and its influence around the British Isles. Sadly, that early, inspiring center is no longer in operation. However, its partner-training model can still be felt in some British Health Regions, as well as in research conducted at City University, London. It is also gratifying to know that in 2016, Re-Connect opened its doors in Southwark, under the capable direction of Sally McVicker, and at other locations in London. The goals at Re-Connect are shared with other aphasia centers and groups across the English-speaking world. Essentially, they are to help individuals and families get on with life, participate in society once again, and to share the camaraderie that infuses aphasia groups and centers everywhere.

Moving on to Australia, it was my great good luck to have met Linda Worrall from the University of Queensland, in Brisbane, and at an Academy of Aphasia meeting in Boston in the late 1980s. She came to visit briefly in Pittsburgh the next year, and soon after, I moved to the University of Arizona, and Linda came for a longer stay. Thus began one of the richest experiences of my life in aphasia. I learned more from Linda and her doctoral student, Madeline Cruice, now at the City, University of London, who also put in some research time in Tucson, than they ever learned from me. And due to the trips that followed, when I was a Visiting Professor at the Universities of Queensland and Sydney, and then at Edith Cowan University in Perth, I had the joy of learning from many of the major figures in the world of aphasia and related disciplines there. These included (among many others) Miranda Rose, Elizabeth Armstrong, Leanne Togher, and Deborah Hersh. Perhaps, there is something in the freshness and energy of life "down under" that breeds the freshness and energy of their preeminent and continuing contributions to the growth of the Social Imperative.

Linda Worrall retired in 2019. Many of her colleagues participated in writing a comprehensive summary of her boundless contributions to the Social Imperative to aphasia worldwide (Wallace et al., 2019). A paraphrase from their abstract summarizes her influence almost too succinctly: "Research capacity building and implementation of clinical aphasia research about aphasia, and improvement of emotional outcomes of aphasia, Linda Worrall's work has had great reach across the English-speaking world" (p. 88).

Canada was left for last on this international tour of English-speaking influences on my version of history of the Social Imperative in the United States. Aura Kagan arrived in Toronto and joined forces with Pat Arato, sometime in the early to mid-1980s. I wish I had been there to watch what must have been their instantaneous recognition of meeting a soulmate. Under Aura Kagan's masterful leadership, the Aphasia Center of North York grew into The Aphasia Institute, probably the most respected aphasia resource in the world, not only for those fortunate to attend it, but because of its training programs for clinicians worldwide, and its vast catalog of clinical resources for use by other centers. I suspect that in at least one of these forms, the Aphasia Institute has influenced almost all of the aphasia clinics and centers in the Western world.

Scurrying on to another "When Harry Met Sally" of the Social Imperative movement, it must have occurred "When Aura met Nina" (Simmons-Mackie) in the 1980s. Their professional collaboration has been one of the most productive in the contemporary history of aphasia. More on this later.

The Nineties, and Dribbling Over into the 21st Century

Pelagie Beeson and I began our university-centered Aphasia Clinic soon after I arrived in Tucson in 1991. Although I was no stranger to group treatment, our Arizona clinic gave me my chance to do it essentially (Pagie's) and my way. Because we ran our aphasia group program as part of our roles in the newly funded National Center for Neurogenic Communication Disorders, it served to recruit individuals to be part of our research endeavors. It also satisfied my longing to be involved in group treatment of aphasia.

Although not exactly household words, "aphasia groups" were forming in academic and social settings, such as churches,

YMCAs, hospitals, and so forth, across the United States. Their founders included dedicated families, volunteers, centers for aging, and clinicians who had caught the Social Imperative bug. Some were purely social, some provided aphasia group therapy, and some had mixed agendas. But there they were. I suspect in almost all cases, they brought smiles to the faces of people with aphasia, grateful for spouses who could talk to each other and be freed from their caregiver responsibilities for a bit of time, and everybody (including clinicians) began to feel a bit safer with their new knowledge that they were not alone in their interests in aphasia's social consequences. One of the most important voices in this movement was that of Jon Lyon whose work in training conversational and interactional partners (Lyon, 1989, 1992) set the stage for much that was to follow.

Roberta Elman, another mover and shaker, founded the Aphasia Center of California in 1996 as the first independent nonprofit organization in the United States dedicated to providing community-based services related to the consequences of aphasia for PWA and their significant others. The creation of the Aphasia Center of California followed completion of Elman and Bernstein-Ellis' randomized controlled trial that had investigated the efficacy of aphasia groups for individuals with chronic aphasia. The publication of this seminal research (Elman & Bernstein-Ellis, 1999) was critical to furthering the Social Imperative, as was the first edition of Elman's book on neurogenic treatment groups (Elman, 1999). Following publication of the study and the book, Roberta has made it her life mission to share information about Life Participation Approach to Aphasia (LPAA) and aphasia group treatment at continuing education venues around the world.

Quoting oneself is probably bad form, but I think I caught the temper of the times in my forward to Simmons-Mackie, King, and Beukelman's comprehensive text *Supporting Communication for Adults with Acute and Chronic Aphasia* (2013). I described the 1990s as the time when "modest warfare" began regarding the treatment of aphasia. Central to the skirmishes was the World Health Organization's dichotomization (as published in 2001) of the "impairment of aphasia (as well as many other impairments) from their effects, that is, its consequences." For aphasia, "consequences" meant that the disorder constrained everyday functioning and restricted the aphasic speaker's ability to return to his or her previous roles in everyday communicative life. Of course, it is not necessary to swear loyalty to an impairment or even to a consequences model as defined in this way. However, minor skirmishes did break out, and for many clinicians and researchers, it grew increasingly difficult to maintain neutrality.

2000–2010

By 2000, the skirmishes intensified, and a group of visionary clinicians (Roberta Chapey, Judith Duchan, Roberta Elman, Linda Garcia, Aura Kagan, Jon Lyon, and Nina Simmons-Mackie) decided they had had it with life participation being ignored by many aphasiologists at the same time as swallowing therapy was pushing aphasia treatment to the curb. They stepped forward with a document entitled *Life Participation Approach to Aphasia: A Statement of Values for the Future* (LPAA Project Group, 2000). It is a "call to arms" about bringing real world concerns quite explicitly into aphasia treatment. To remind readers of the LPAA statement of the five core principles, here they are:

1. The explicit goal is the enhancement of life participation.
2. Everyone affected by aphasia is entitled to service.
3. Success measures include documented life enhancement changes.
4. Both personal and environmental factors are intervention targets.
5. Emphasis is on availability of services as needed at all stages of aphasia.

I could only scream "YES! YES! YES!" when I read it. I felt like chains had been removed, that the message was floating in big cloud formations all over the Arizona sky; I felt free to be clinical me, not abandoning impairment work, but freeing me to confront the whole complex picture of aphasia and what I could do to help to minimize aphasia's effect on getting on with life as fully and as quickly as possible. In my view, the LPAA statement was the catalyst that, in the United States, led to the proliferation of aphasia groups and the growth of more comprehensive aphasia centers.

By now, the forerunner to Connect was up and running at City, University of London, by 1995 with Sally Byng as its leader, and with its activities well described in *Beyond Aphasia* (Pound, Parr, Lindsay, & Woolf, 2000). Nevertheless, the opening of Aphasia Connect in 2001 in London was a tipping point. Soon Connect was not alone; it was influencing the whole English-speaking world.

I was fortunate to be at Aura Kagan's incredibly innovative talk "Supported Conversation in Aphasia" at the Clinical Aphasiology Conference meeting in Sedona in 1993. It was a landmark event, startlingly simple, gobsmacking, making the conference participants consider why nobody before Aura had figured out the glaringly obvious importance training *nonaphasic people* in how to encourage, reinforce, and support the speaking efforts of PWA. To me, it was a turning point, and with its publication (1998), its influence on the Social Imperative was huge. It remains a cornerstone for clinicians, and for me, required reading for any neophyte clinician interested in the Social Imperative in Aphasia.

I don't know when and how "Nina met Aura" but they were both authors of the LPAA statement, so it had to be before 2000. Regardless, that meeting of minds has had immense effects on the Social Imperative in Aphasia. They are responsible for Aphasia-Framework for Outcome Measurement (A-FROM) (Kagan et al., 2008) the theoretical basis for the Assessment for Living with Aphasia (ALA) (Simmons-Mackie et al., 2014). Kagan and Simmons-Mackie have had a long history of cooperative work and lecturing that has altered the face of North American aphasiology.

The Adler Aphasia Center in Maywood, New Jersey opened in 2003. I am sure I can't name them all, but a number of aphasia centers include the Houston Aphasia Recovery Center (HARC), the Aphasia Center of West Texas, the program at the (then) Rehabilitation Institute of Chicago, the Triangle Aphasia Project (TAP) in North Carolina, the Stroke Comeback Center, and the Snyder Center for Aphasia Life Enhancement (SCALE) in Baltimore. all opened before 2010. And, to the best of my knowledge, the first private practice that centered on life participation and aphasia was "Speaking of Aphasia" founded in 2004 by Shirley Morganstein and Marilyn Certner Smith.

My more recent history is really tied up in the Adler Aphasia Center. Not surprisingly, few psychosocial services were available to Mike Adler after he suffered an aphasia/apraxia-producing stroke and was discharged from traditional aphasia therapy. Was it that way all across the English-speaking world? Mike and Elaine his wife, knowing how to get things done, hired an investigative reporter to find out what was available in the English-speaking world. The resultant comprehensive and accurate report resulted in their decision to visit Centers in (surprise!) Toronto, Ontario, Canada, London, United Kingdom, and Oakland, California, as well as our program at the University of Arizona. Little did I know that I was being interviewed for a part time job, but soon thereafter, they invited me to come and help them with their decision to do an aphasia center in Maywood, New Jersey, and to sign on as its research director. When the doors opened perhaps six months later, the Adler Center was almost immediately successful in serving the needs of PWA and their families in New York and New Jersey.

A few years later, Mike and Elaine wanted to encourage the development of Adler-like aphasia centers across the country. The needs of people in Oakland, California, for example, were well served by the Aphasia Center of California, and likewise, the Aphasia Institute's goals and programs were shaped by the needs of their Toronto members, so I politely begged to disagree. Hometown interests topped generic concerns. Karen Tucker, the Adler Center Director and I convinced Mike and Elaine to sponsor a meeting for representatives from existing Centers to get together and discuss their mutual concerns, frustrations, and successes and to take a look at their diversity and indigenous roots. That meeting occurred in New Jersey in 2011.

I was privileged to attend this, the best meeting I ever went to. All 28 or so persons in attendance, representing 17 North American aphasia programs, learned about others' solutions to mutual problems. They also shared their activities and programs that really worked, and what appeared to be great ideas that bombed. It was clear by the end of the meeting that this group needed to meet again, enhanced by the new centers that continued to pop up.

The Aphasia Center of West Texas agreed to help with underwriting the expenses of the second meeting, and in 2013, we reconvened. The same enthusiasm was there, along with new ideas and new blood, and increasing good fellowship. By the end of an almost-three-day meeting in Midland, Texas, Liz Hoover from Boston University declared that "we needed to grow and keep going."

We had no money, but we were full of enthusiasm and energy. With all of that going for us, we decided to become a national group. The following winter (2013), a small group convened in Santa Fe and in two days wrote the structure and by-laws for what we decided to term "Aphasia Access." In 2014, Aphasia Access became an official nonprofit organization and began as a "Coordinated mechanism for sharing information, solving challenges and helping new providers . . . (it is) a network of health care, business, and community leaders to advance lifelong communication access for people with aphasia." The first large biannual meeting was held in Boston in 2015, the second in Orlando in 2017, and in 2019, Aphasia Access held its third National meeting in Baltimore. All three meetings displayed a camaraderie unique to people whose ideas and values mesh. Those meetings seemed to me to be Aphasia's Woodstock, with good fellowship being a worthy substitute for drugs.

Aphasia Access membership currently comprises over 300 aphasia programs, practicing clinicians, graduate students, educators, and administrators. New centers and groups have begun. A classroom module is available to instructors to introduce the movement. The module can be plugged into ongoing academic courses in aphasia taught to prospective clinicians. Simmons-Mackie's comprehensive publication (2018) on the status of aphasia in North America is available through Aphasia Access. Frequent informative presentations are available via Aphasia Access for members who are uncertain about how to move beyond training in impairment-based to consequence-based approaches to aphasia management, and a fascinating series of lectures and interviews is available online.

The online presence of Aphasia Access leads well into what I believe might be a paradigm shift toward the Social Imperative in the United States. Perhaps because so few graduate training programs include a substantial focus on it, a growing trend over the past 20 or so years has been the growth not only of online resources for clinicians who wish to learn more about social issues and useful intervention approaches, but also the growing popularity of hands-on workshops taught by its major practitioners. In this regard, both Roberta Elman and Maura Silverman of TAP could well be considered the Johanna Appleseeds of the Social Imperative Movement. National and state meetings hold overflow sessions and an online webinar has even provided the impetus for this book. There is something so socially right about all of that!

Onward . . . Aphasia Meets the Next 50 Years of the Social Imperative

The scope of activities is clearly vibrant, alive, and well. There are also exciting additions on the horizon. This movement must take advantage of technological advancement, not only in relation to impairment-focused drills, but also extending the reach of the multifaceted media into contributions to the Social Imperative. The Aphasia Recovery Connection (ARC) is a remarkable, successful Internet group that permits PWA and their families to meet, discuss problems, and communicate with like others, no matter where they are. It is a marvelous prototype. Carol Dow-Richards and her son David who, as a child had an adult-like aphasia and has relatively mild but still improving aphasia for 25 years, can be jointly credited for recognizing the power of the Internet in serving a wide slice of the aphasia world, much of which is unable to attend centers and groups for myriad reasons, such as health, distance to programs, lack of transportation, and so forth. But the Dows have not stopped there. The ARC also arranges events for people with neurogenic disorders and their families to simply learn and enjoy in the presence of like others. Aphasia Boot Camps, cruises, and such, are the result. I feel confident that services currently online to help individuals with aphasia with impairment-focused activities will continue to expand to meet the Social Imperative over the next few years. Their developers are aware of the bigger truth: Internet-focused services are just the starting point for moving from impairment-oriented drills to even better services that meet long-term communicative needs. We are not there yet, but "oh the progress is great . . . "

Closing Thoughts

After Martha Sarno, I believe I am one of the first persons to have bought into the movement here in the United States. I wish the Social Imperative had gained traction earlier. It might have had more significant impact on health care delivery had it excited more people earlier. That didn't happen, but the movement is clearly growing now and there is little doubt that treatment for the long-term consequences of aphasia is respected and valued. It has been a wonderful ride. I have been privileged to observe and participate in changes and in growth of truly remarkable and innovative ideas. I believe that our profession has become much better at serving aphasic individuals with chronic aphasia and their loved ones. More slowly, perhaps more subtly, this spirit has begun to influence some other neurogenic speech and language disorders that our profession serves. I believe this book adequately reflects some of these changes as well.

I am still bothered, however, by the fact that so few training programs in this country go beyond the traditional anatomy and neurobiology of language and treating its impairments, to include the bigger issues of how these disorders destroy or minimize quality of life, and what we can do about THAT! In my opinion, our idealistic, dedicated students have to be prepared to become part of the solution, rather than to have their training focus on being part of the problem.

I am basically a happy person. I have always loved my work in research and in interacting with resilient brave people and families with aphasia. But I think that after family (including my animals), what has contributed most consistently to my personal happiness has been fellowship with like-minded professionals who always seem to be there for me, the joy of teaching, my research buddies and collaborators, my wonderful students, and again, the people with aphasia and their families with whom I have been privileged to know and to work with. I am unwilling to single out any of them, particularly when there is a page limit to this chapter—there are just too many to whom I am indebted for making my career so fulfilling. Students, many collaborators, families, and people with aphasia, they have in large measure made my life complete. Please understand why I have limited my acknowledgements so rigidly.

Finally, I previously noted that I have been coming to the Adler Aphasia Center since its inception. Whenever I go there, I am struck by the noise, the laughter, the industriousness, and the pervasive good fellowship of these persons with aphasia, their staff, volunteers, and their loved ones. Some of the Center's original staff and members have been coming to Adler as long as I have. When I show up, the member old timers treat me as if I am a long lost cousin. In essence, I go to the Adler Center to be validated. That is at the heart of the Social Imperative. But, isn't there also something kind of backward in that? Who should be validating whom?

References

Austin, J. L. (1975). *How to do things with words*. Cambridge, MA: Harvard University Press.

Bates, E. (1976). *Language and context: The acquisition of pragmatics*. New York, NY: Academic Press.

Benton, A., & Joynt, R. J. (1960). Early descriptions of aphasia. *Archives of Neurology, 3*, 205–222. PMID137990043. doi10.1001/archneur,19600450020085012

Dick, F., Bates, E., Wulfeck, B., Utman, J. A., Dronkers, N., & Gernsbacher, M. A. (2001). Language deficits, localization, and grammar: Evidence for a distributive model of language breakdown in aphasic patients and neurologically intact individuals. *Psychological Review, 108*(4), 759.

Elman, R. (Ed.). (1999). *Group treatment of neurogenic communication disorders: The expert clinician's approach*. Boston, MA: Butterworth.

Elman, R., & Bernstein-Ellis, E. (1999). The efficacy of group communication treatment in adults with chronic aphasia. *Journal of Speech Language and Hearing Research, 42*(2),411–419. https://doi.org/10.1044/jslhr.4202.411

Fromm, D., Forbes, M., Holland, A., & MacWhinney, B. (2020). Using AphasiaBank for discourse assessment. *Seminars in Speech and Language, 41*, 10–19. https://doi.org/10.1055/s-0039-3399499

Grice, P. (1975). Logic and conversation. In P. Cole & J. Morgan (Eds.), *Syntax and semantics, 3: Speech acts* (pp. 41–58). New York, NY: Academic Press.

Holland, A., Fromm, D., & Wozniak, L. (2018). *Communicative activities of daily living* (3rd ed.). Austin, TX: Pro-Ed.

Kagan, A. (1998). Supported conversation for adults with aphasia: Methods and resources for training conversation partners, *Aphasiology, 12*(9), 816–830. https://doi.org/10.1080/0268703980824957

Kagan, A., Simmons-Mackie, N., Rowland, A., Huijbregts, M., Shumway, E., McEwen, S., . . . Sharp, S. (2008). Counting what counts: A framework for capturing real-life outcomes of aphasia intervention. *Aphasiology, 22*(3), 258–280. https://doi.org/10.1080/02687030701282595

Kagan, A., & Gailey, G. (1993). Functional is not enough. In A. Holland & M. Forbes (Eds.), *Aphasia treatment: World perspectives*. San Diego, CA: Singular Publishing

LPAA Project Group. (2000). Life participation approach to aphasia: A statement of values for the future. *ASHA Leader, 5*(3), 4–6. Retrieved from https://www.asha.org/public/speech/disorders/LPAA .htm Reprinted in R. Chapey (2001) (Ed.), *Language intervention strategies in aphasia and related neurogenic communication disorders* (4th ed.). Baltimore, MD: Lippincott, Williams & Wilkins.

Lyon, J. (1989). Communication partners: Their value in reestablishing communication with aphasic adults. In T. Prescott (Ed.), *Clinical aphasiology conference proceedings* (Vol. 18, pp. 11–17). Boston, MA: College-Hill Press.

Lyon, J. (1992). Communicative use and participation in life for aphasic adults in natural settings: The scope of the problem. *American Journal of Speech and Language Pathology, 1*(3), 7–14.

Penn, C. (1993). Aphasia therapy in South Africa: Some pragmatic and personal perspectives. In A. Holland & M. Forbes, M. (Eds.), *Aphasia treatment: World perspectives*. San Diego, CA: Singular Publishing.

Pound, C., Parr, S., Lindsay, J., & Woolf, C. (2000). *Beyond aphasia: Therapies for living with communication disability*. Oxon, UK: Winslow Press.

Sarno, M. T. (1969). *The functional communication profile: Manual of directions*. Rehabilitation Monograph 42, New York Medical Center, New York, NY.

Searle, J. (1969). *Speech acts: An essay in the philosophy of language*. Cambridge, UK: University Press.

Simmons-Mackie, N. (2018). *Aphasia in North America: Frequency, demographics, impact of aphasia. Communication access, services and service gaps*. Available at http://www.aphasiaaccess.org

Simmons-Mackie, N., Kagan, A., Victor, J. C., Carling-Rowland, A., Mok, A., Hoch, J. S., . . . Streiner, D. L. (2014). The assessment for living with aphasia: Reliability and construct validity. *International Journal of Speech-Language Pathology, 16*(1), 82–94.

Simmons-Mackie, N., King, J. M., & Beukelman, D. R. (Eds.). (2013). *Supporting communication for adults with acute and chronic aphasia.* Towson, MD: Brookes.

Wallace, S. J., Baker, C., Brandenburg, C., Bryant, L., Le Dorze, G., Power, E., & Shrubsole, K. (2019). A how-to guide to aphasia services: Celebrating Professor Linda Worrall's contribution to the field. *Aphasiology, 33*(7), 888–902.

Watzlawick, J., Beavin, J., & Jackson, D. (1967). *Pragmatics of human communication.* New York, NY: W. W. Norton.

Wepman, J. (1951). *Recovery from aphasia.* New York, NY: Ronald Press.

World Health Organization (2001). *International classification of function, disability, and health.* Geneva, Switzerland: Author.

C.A.P.E.

A CHECKLIST OF FOUR ESSENTIAL AND EVIDENCE-BASED CATEGORIES FOR APHASIA INTERVENTION

Roberta J. Elman

Reaching for C.A.P.E.: A Personal Evolution Toward the Social Imperative

As a master's degree student at the University of Minnesota, I was thrilled when I was finally provided the opportunity to work with adult clients who were living with communication disorders, especially aphasia. I was enthusiastic to learn as much as I could about the disorders they had acquired. I found myself reading, and then rereading, my course notes, and checking out every textbook that I could find in the library that discussed aphasia treatment. The goal I set for myself was to find the right aphasia treatment or technique that could fix the impaired speech and language skills, to help these individuals regain their lives.

I began to realize in Minnesota, and also especially during my Clinical Fellowship (CF) position in Eugene, Oregon, that I was failing. One of my Oregon clients, Rose, drove with her husband almost an hour one way for her twice weekly sessions with me at the Hearing and Speech Center. Her stroke had left her with a severe Broca's aphasia and coexisting apraxia of speech. She was able to produce a few words as well as an occasional social greeting, but not much else. I dove into Rose's therapy with utter enthusiasm, using interventions such as tasks involving intonation and singing, apraxia of speech drills, and treatments focused on language stimulation. And after more than six months of treatment, it became apparent that progress outside the therapy room was minimal. There were gains documented on some standardized tests, but little had transferred to life with her husband. Rose was discouraged. And so was I. Why hadn't I discovered the right way to unlock her speech and language skills? Was it my therapy? Was it me?

When my CF ended in 1982, I moved to San Diego to accept a position at a medical rehabilitation program that was part of a large hospital. My outpatient caseload consisted entirely of adults who had survived either a traumatic brain injury or a stroke. I was particularly drawn to the individuals who were living with aphasia. They were so motivated to regain their communication skills. I believed that in this "state of the art" environment, I would be able to find ways to "fix" them. I remember Ted, a gentleman who has sustained a stroke with resulting aphasia about one month prior. He had retired from his job just three months before his stroke. Ted and his wife had made plans to take a series of vacations to visit all the places they had always wanted to see. Instead, Ted was coming to the rehabilitation center three times a week, receiving speech, physical, and occupational therapies. He was motivated to improve and worked tirelessly on the tasks in my treatment room and also on the homework sheets that I sent home with him each session. I worked with Ted for more than a year. And I failed him, too.

I had concentrated on general language stimulation tasks across the language modalities, including using repetition and cloze techniques. "Up and _____." "Right and _____." I had individualized a set of purchased data sheets, popular at the time, for keeping scores for every item during each session. I could demonstrate some improvement over time on these tasks, and also on the standardized aphasia tests I repeatedly administered. But Ted's communication hadn't improved much at home. And he was too stigmatized by his aphasia to get back to doing things in the community with friends or family members. And I'm sorry to say, that providing him with communication supports to help him resume some of these interests, didn't occur to me.

I did have a couple of isolated successes with two other clients who were living with aphasia. But I can't really claim full credit for those successes. One client, Jean, had been trying hard to explain something to her husband. But her language skills weren't up to the task. And that was especially true because she hadn't received any communication supports from me or anyone else. It was tax time and she had been the one who had completed their taxes before her stroke. Jean and her husband were both frustrated. And for some reason, I grabbed a pad of paper and a pen, and we worked together to see if she could draw a picture that might transmit some information. And she actually did! She drew a fairly good sketch of an oil derrick, and when her husband saw it, he remembered that he needed to include the revenue from an oil investment in their tax returns. There were smiles all around. I would be lying if I told you that this success led to my trying communicative drawing in my therapy routinely going forward. But this wouldn't happen for another four or five years.

A brilliant woman, Betty, who had been living with Wernicke's aphasia for two months, tried repeatedly to teach me some important lessons. But at that time, I didn't have the right theoretical framework to learn those lessons from her. Betty lived in an upscale assisted living community in San Diego and ordered her meals every day in the dining room. She had become frustrated when the wait staff came to take her order, because the paraphasias and neologisms she produced weren't understood. However, Betty had traveled the world. And she realized that she could bring a Berlitz travel book that she had in her apartment to the community dining room. Because her reading for words and phrases was quite good, she was able to use the Berlitz book to point to various menu items that were listed. And when this was successful, she was excited to let me know. She brought her Berlitz book to our therapy session one day and I was fascinated at both her ingenuity and the technique. But it would be several years before I would think about trying something similar with other individuals who had aphasia.

Betty and I always spent the first 10 minutes of each session in conversation. She wanted so much to talk to someone! She used a number of effective strategies without training, and with gestures, a little writing, and some pantomime, as well as the questions that I asked, we were able to have some amazing conversations on such topics as eastern philosophy and national politics. Betty was interested in so many things and, looking back, I bet that those 10 minutes at the beginning of each session was the only time she really engaged in conversation with anyone. But I felt so guilty taking 10 minutes away from each session for conversation, even if we were using strategies, because, in my mind, it didn't "qualify" as therapy. At least what I had been taught was therapy. Instead, I thought that we needed to move on to the various structured therapy tasks that I had created on the data sheets.

I was disillusioned. How come I couldn't fix aphasia? I knew I must have been doing something wrong because these failures had never been discussed in the courses I had taken, the textbooks I was reading, or during any discussions with my clinical supervisors. So my answer was to go back to school and learn more. I enrolled in the Speech and Hearing Sciences doctoral program at the University of California, Santa Barbara. I was still looking for a key that could unlock the communication skills of the people I was working with—people who were living with aphasia. I actually had some sense that creating a Stroke Center could provide an answer. And I put that thought on the back burner as I packed up and headed up the coast of California.

I gained a lot of knowledge in my coursework. But it was mainly due to the influence of my doctoral advisor, the late Carol Prutting, that my doctoral studies were special. Her support, encouragement, good humor, and wisdom were worth all of the challenges that came with being a doctoral student. Importantly, Carol's area was pragmatics, specifically in child language acquisition, and we had had some discussions about how work in sociolinguistics might inform the study of aphasia. But these ideas were at a conceptual level, and my doctoral program didn't provide the time I needed for thinking more about this. In 1986, I was ready to begin collecting data for my dissertation—its focus was on cueing and priming of naming in aphasia. I once again packed my belongings and headed up the coast of California, this time landing in the San Francisco Bay Area. There, I had a wonderful opportunity to learn from talented colleagues at the Martinez VA while completing my dissertation research.

But it was actually a conference that changed my professional world. I submitted a paper to the 1988 Clinical Aphasiology Conference. The conference was held in Cape Cod that year and I attended knowing few people there. One person I knew was my "boss" at the Martinez VA, Terry Wertz. When I arrived at the conference, he immediately introduced me to Audrey Holland. That was thrilling! And, when the conference began, I heard three incredible papers. The first was presented by Nina Simmons-Mackie. She discussed "Easy Street"—a life-size re-creation of a shopping street from a prototypical small town. Easy Street helped clients practice language skills in everyday activities. Immediately, I began nodding my head. I knew that is what Betty, Rose, Ted, and Jean had needed. Practice with everyday language. Then Jon Lyon presented two thought provoking papers. One discussed "Communicative Partners" and the other "Communicative Drawing." My head nodding must have looked pathologic at this point! But in those first 48 hours, I had met three aphasiologists who would change the direction of my career. And, once we met one another, we were off on a journey that led to the push for acceptance of a social model, and articulation of the Life Participation Approach to Aphasia (LPAA; LPAA Project Group, 2000).

After the 1988 CAC, I had the opportunity to travel to Toronto for a conference sponsored by the Speech and Stroke Centre —North York (now known as the Aphasia Institute). Jon Lyon had suggested that I attend the conference and also visit their aphasia program directed by Aura Kagan. Visiting the Centre in September 1989, and getting to know Aura, was another turning point in my career. During my time there, I was able to observe a number of different aphasia groups that were facilitated by volunteers. That day of observation convinced me that group therapy held real promise for improving the communication skills of people living with aphasia. I vowed to find a way to research the efficacy of aphasia group treatment. My personal evolution toward embracing a social imperative for aphasia intervention was on its way. I finished my doctoral program in 1990 and accepted a position as head of a speech-language pathology department at an Easter Seals outpatient medical rehabilitation center. Now I just needed to figure out a way to address my research interest in aphasia group therapy and spend some time musing about the Stroke Center idea that I had while working in San Diego.

Often when you see people at conferences, you may have a wonderful conversation or two, and promise to keep in touch, but then you return to your own work environment and don't seem to connect with them again until a year later, at the next conference. But the small group of us that met in 1988 and 1989 did stay connected. We were so excited about the prospect of bringing a social approach into the field of aphasiology that we scheduled conference calls and planned meetings before and after ASHA conventions or CAC meetings. We were frustrated that the increasing focus on treatment for swallowing disorders was resulting in people with aphasia not receiving services for their language disorder. We were also frustrated that some of our own aphasiology colleagues didn't seem to appreciate the need for a social model. Looking back, I think we were equal parts passionate and naive. We knew that there was a need for a paradigm shift, and somehow concluded that we were the ones to make that change happen.

While working at Easter Seals, I discovered that the National Easter Seal Society had a grant program to fund rehabilitative research. A grant that I wrote to investigate the efficacy of aphasia group treatment for individuals with chronic aphasia was funded in 1994. Ellen Bernstein-Ellis and I would spend the next two years working on this project. Our randomized controlled trial demonstrated that people with chronic aphasia made statistically significant changes on standardized measures of both language and communication. But the information we gathered from our qualitative interviews was the big surprise. We found that participants had made gains that had transferred into the community and well beyond the conversational tasks that we had focused on during treatment (Elman & Bernstein-Ellis, 1999a, 1999b). Family members shared that some participants were now ordering for themselves at restaurants, taking back shoes that didn't fit, and feeling confident enough to take a trip on a motorcycle that had been in storage since the stroke. Importantly, participants and family members reported that there had been numerous psychosocial benefits from participating in the groups (Elman & Bernstein-Ellis, 1999b). These were the types of outcomes that I had been trying to achieve for years! And the results of the study catapulted me straight into unchartered territory. In 1996, I resigned my position at Easter Seals and volunteered my time for the next three years to create the infrastructure and programming at the Aphasia Center of California. With Ellen Bernstein-Ellis and Sue Ewing helping with facilitating the aphasia groups, I could spend time on developing a sustainable service delivery model that was outside third-party payers/managed care. My personal evolution toward embracing a social approach for aphasia intervention was complete. Now the challenge was in trying to build a community of like-minded professionals.

As I was starting the Aphasia Center of California, I continued to believe that there hadn't been enough progress made with shifting aphasia intervention in the direction of a social imperative. And those of us who were trying to do work within a social model were getting a number of rejections, from both publications and conferences. So, I suggested that we hold our own small conference where participants could each present work aligned with the social model. We wanted to allow ample time for discussion as well as informal interactions. We called this meeting "Non-Traditional Approaches to Aphasia" and it was held in Yountville, California in March 1997. We had hoped that there might be a dozen or so people interested in attending. Honestly, we were concerned that the meeting might not attract enough interest. However, interest was much higher than we ever anticipated, and because we wanted to prioritize interactions among participants, we capped attendance at 22 people. Participants came from across the U.S., Canada, and England. This conference was successful in many ways. It provided a supportive venue for people to exchange ideas. It also resulted in future meetings and collaborations. Several smaller meetings followed, including a Martha's Vineyard meeting in 1998, a meeting in Dorset, England in 2001 hosted by Sally Byng, Susie Parr, and Carole Pound, and a meeting in Toronto, Canada, hosted by Aura Kagan in 2007. Importantly, a group of seven attendees from the Martha's Vineyard meeting decided to form the Life Participation Approach to Aphasia Project group (alphabetically: Roberta Chapey, Judith Duchan, Roberta Elman, Linda Garcia, Aura Kagan, Jon Lyon, and Nina Simmons-Mackie) with the purpose of publishing a position paper to move the cause forward. A series of conference calls and e-mails, as well as more than a few passionate discussions, resulted in a document that we could all support; our LPAA position paper was published in the ASHA Leader in 2000 (LPAA Project Group, 2000).

Life Participation Approach to Aphasia

Building on the work of such aphasiology pioneers as Martha Taylor Sarno and Audrey Holland, LPAA is a philosophy that emphasizes reengagement in life for all those affected by aphasia (LPAA Project Group, 2000). LPAA's foundation was derived from a number of theoretical concepts and frameworks, including the World Health Organization's International Classification of Functioning, Disability, and Health (ICF), which integrates medical and social models (WHO, 2001). LPAA attempts to unite a variety of approaches to assessment, intervention, research, and advocacy with five core components in its framework: (1) The explicit goal is enhancement of life participation. (2) All those affected by aphasia are entitled to service. (3) Both personal and environmental factors are targets of assessment and intervention. (4) Success is measured via documented life enhancement changes. (5) Emphasis is placed on availability of services as needed at all stages of life with aphasia. LPAA suggests that advocacy efforts should be targeted to those components that are not available in our current health care systems. You can read the original LPAA position paper that has been reprinted in the Prologue of this book. This version includes a table of clinical examples and a short list of the original references. The full set of references from the original article are available on the Aphasia Institute's website (http://www.aphasia.ca).

Finding C.A.P.E.

Working at the Aphasia Center of California (ACC) has been my dream come true. I have had the opportunity to meet amazing people who are living with aphasia, as well as talented SLPs who have become part of our ACC community. Each person with aphasia, as a member of one or more aphasia groups, and with the guidance of a speech-language pathologist facilitator, provides support and suggestions to the other group members. The power of the group is that each person with aphasia learns from the others. People find out about the ACC in a variety of ways. Some are referred by speech-language pathologists or other health care professionals in the Northern California Bay Area. Others hear about us from friends and family members who find us via "word of mouth" or have located information about the ACC during an internet search. Some new group members have been living with aphasia for weeks, others for years.

Over the last decade, I began to notice that more and more PWA were arriving at the ACC unable to use any strategies for communication, either with or without family members or friends. In addition, many PWA and family members told us that they hadn't received education about aphasia from health care providers. These seemed like changes and were definite challenges for the SLPs at the ACC. Our conversation groups hadn't been developed to teach "basic" communication skills. Instead, we wanted to build on the basic skills that clients had received in individual treatment before coming to our program.

I believe that an increasing demand for productivity across clinical care settings is impacting the type of treatment that PWA and their family members are currently receiving. The increased demand for productivity naturally results in less time for treatment planning. This also results in a tendency for SLPs to pull a workbook from a shelf or open a computerized app instead of taking some time to discover what communication strategies are most effective for that individual. I also realized that many professional workshops and book chapters were providing therapists with a wide array of aphasia treatments, but not providing a sense of priorities.

So, in order to help you think more about clinical priorities, I am going to provide you with a frightening scenario. I would like each of you reading this chapter to take a few minutes to think about the scenario below and to write down your answers. We'll come back to those a bit later:

- What if tomorrow **you** had a stroke with moderate to severe aphasia?
- Your medical insurance will authorize a total of 16 sessions for your SLP to work with you.
- You will not receive any additional speech-language therapy after these 16 sessions have been completed.
- What would you like your speech-language pathologist to focus on in the 16 sessions that have been authorized for you?

My goal was to develop a checklist that could help SLPs focus on treatment essentials. Fewer sessions authorized for aphasia treatment mean that we must make every session count. Each session is precious to that person and family and time shouldn't be wasted on treatments that are unlikely to benefit *that* person or *that* family. Clinicians should not be pulling a workbook (or an app) from the shelf just as the PWA walks into the room. My "Aphasia Treatment Essentials" checklist became what is known as C.A.P.E. (Elman, 2013, 2016, 2018a, 2018b):

C: Connecting People with Aphasia

A: Augmentative & Alternative Communication

P: Partner Training

E: Education & Resources

Now, thinking back to the scenario I gave you above, if **you** had a stroke and were living with moderate or severe aphasia, did you want your SLP to work on some of the categories listed on the C.A.P.E. checklist? Perhaps you wanted to be able to communicate with your family, friends, or health care professionals? Or maybe you wanted to learn more about aphasia and the other resources available in your community, including where you could meet others living with aphasia?

Some of the C.A.P.E. treatment essentials are most appropriate for those with a moderate or severe level of aphasia. Other treatment essentials are appropriate for anyone affected by aphasia. Note that these categories are not prescriptive or exhaustive. They simply serve as a clinical "high priority" checklist, especially during the first few months of aphasia intervention. These suggested treatment categories are all evidence-based and they were selected based on research about what people with aphasia, their family members, and their friends wished they had received in the first few months of treatment (Aphasia United Best Practice Statements, n.d.; Avent et al., 2005; Brown, Worrall, Davidson, & Howe, 2012; Elman, Cohen, & Silverman, 2016; Hilton, Leenhouts, Webster, & Morris, 2014; Hinckley, Hasselkus, & Ganzfried, 2013; Howe et al., 2012; Parr, Byng, Gilpin, & Ireland, 1997; Power et al., 2015; Wallace et al., 2017; Worrall et al., 2011). These categories were also based on my own clinical observations gathered over more than thirty years of working with thousands of people with aphasia. In addition, a survey of caregivers of PWA collected in the western and mid-Atlantic regions of the United States validated that many families and PWA are not receiving these treatment essentials (Elman et al., 2016).

The next sections provide some additional information and examples for each category on the C.A.P.E. checklist. I share a client story at the beginning of each category that is based on real people and events, but I've changed the names and some of the details. The intervention examples I have shared in each category are meant to provide you with some ideas and are not exhaustive. The specific strategies, items, or activities you choose should always be tailored to be personally relevant and meaningful to each individual with aphasia, his/her family, friends, and beyond. When selecting intervention areas and goals with each client, it is helpful to consider all four of the Living with Aphasia: Framework for Outcome Measurement (A-FROM) domains (Kagan et al., 2007). The A-FROM domains were inspired by the ICF (WHO, 2001) Please refer to Figure 2–1.

Living with Aphasia: Framework for Outcome Measurement (A-FROM)

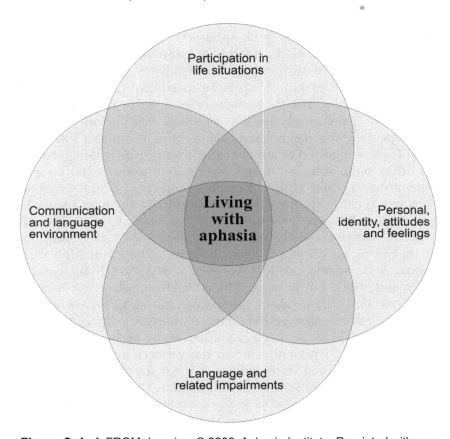

Figure 2–1. A-FROM domains. © 2008, Aphasia Institute. Reprinted with permission of Aphasia Institute.

C.A.P.E. Checklist

C: Connecting People with Aphasia

Why didn't I ever meet other people who had aphasia?

Jack had been living with a moderate Conduction aphasia for more than five years when he walked into the communication group room at the ACC. A family member had called our office after coming across our website. She wondered whether our program might help him. I suggested that Jack sit in on one of the ACC aphasia communication groups the following week. When Jack arrived, he entered the room a bit hesitantly, and then took a seat at the table. He didn't make much eye contact with the SLP or other group members, and didn't say anything at first. But when the SLP asked all the other group members to introduce themselves, as he listened to their names, their backgrounds, and the stories about their stroke and aphasia, you could see his facial expression and posture changing. His head began nodding and a smile crossed his face. And he started to make eye contact. When it was Jack's turn to introduce himself to the others, he said that he had been watching a lot of television since his stroke at the age of 49. He had been an engineer. And he had never met anyone with aphasia until he entered the room that morning. This was true even in a large metropolitan area. You could feel the sense of relief that Jack experienced when he discovered that day that he wasn't all alone . . . more than five years after his stroke with aphasia.

Aphasia is an isolating condition. The language barrier limits access to information about the disorder. This is a decrease in the *transactional* role of language. The language barrier also limits the ability to maintain and create social relationships. This is a decrease in the *interactional* role of language. Many people with aphasia feel that they are all alone—that no one else is living with the disorder. This can cause or exacerbate depression and/or frustration and lead to general psychosocial distress. Meeting other people with aphasia can provide hope and be an important way to see an example of living successfully with aphasia. I also believe that connecting people with aphasia to one another may prevent maladaptive ways of dealing with the disorder.

Few people have heard of aphasia. Studies suggest that only 5% to 10% of the population has a pretty good idea of what it is (Simmons-Mackie, 2018). Even fewer really understand its impact on all aspects of living. This lack of awareness of aphasia, combined with the language barrier that comes with the disorder, presents a huge challenge for the person living with aphasia, family members, friends, and the community at large. There are a variety of ways to connect people with aphasia and I'm going to discuss the following six options:

- Aphasia Groups and Programs
- Communicative Volunteers and Visitation Programs
- Aphasia Conferences
- Aphasia Camps and Cruises
- Meeting Past Clients
- Online Options

I'll be sharing some information about each of them in the following section as well as pointing you to some other resources where you can learn more.

Aphasia Groups and Programs

There has been a rapidly increasing interest in conducting and researching aphasia group therapy since our efficacy study was first published in 1999 (Elman & Bernstein-Ellis, 1999a, 1999b). However, aphasia group therapy actually started during World War II as a way to treat the number of soldiers who were returning home with missile wounds. The field of speech-language pathology was relatively young, and there weren't enough SLPs to provide 1:1 therapy to so many soldiers. Groups provided a solution. In the 1980s, a few studies began to investigate the efficacy and effectiveness of aphasia group treatment (Aten, Caliguiri, & Holland 1982; Bollinger, Musson, & Holland, 1993; Wertz et al, 1981). And since 1999, the number of studies has really blossomed. A full literature review of group therapy is beyond the scope of this chapter, but for those wanting to learn more about aphasia group research, there are a number of chapters, books, journal articles, and webinars that cover this topic (Attard, Lanyon, Togher, & Rose, 2015; Elman, 2007a, 2007b, 2016, 2018a, 2018b, 2018c; Kearns & Elman, 2008; Lanyon, Rose, & Worrall, 2013; Van der Gaag et al., 2005).

I have spent a large portion of my professional career at the ACC working with aphasia groups and have tried to make the research, as well as a variety of clinical and facilitation techniques, available to SLPs. My continuing interest has been in exploring the possible benefits of aphasia group treatment. Here are some of the benefits that I believe can occur in groups:

- Groups promote interaction and variety of communicative functions or speech acts.
- Groups provide opportunity for wider array of partners and therefore may increase the likelihood of generalization.
- Groups promote language improvisation.
- Groups improve psychosocial functioning due to the benefit of community.
- Groups involve more complex language (see Thompson, Shapiro, Kiran, & Sobecks, 2003).
- Groups are cost effective.

Facilitating aphasia groups is complex. Managing the combination of individual and group dynamics requires specific knowledge, skills, and clinical judgment that are best acquired by reading the group treatment literature, as well as gaining appropriate clinical training and supervision. If you are a SLP who wants to start an aphasia group, but you have not received prior education and training, please take the time to read the literature, take advantage of continuing education courses, and consider teaming up with other clinicians who are competent providers of aphasia group therapy (Attard et al., 2015; Bernstein-Ellis & Elman, 2006; Elman, 2007a, 2018a, 2018b, 2020; Ewing, 2007; Kearns & Elman, 2008; Pound, Parr, Lindsay, & Woolf, 2000; Rose & Attard, 2015).

Communicative Volunteers and Visitation Programs

Another way to connect people with aphasia to others is through the use of trained communicative volunteers. Jon Lyon was one of the first aphasiologists to discuss training volunteers in using specific communication strategies with PWA. In Communicative Volunteer programs, volunteers (typically not family members) are recruited and then trained by the SLP on specific communication strategies, methods, and techniques that are effective for that person living with aphasia. Once the SLP determines that the dyad (PWA and volunteer) are communicating well, the PWA chooses some activities to resume or attempt. For example, this might be going to a movie, having lunch at a restaurant, or taking a walk together at a local park. The talk I heard Jon Lyon give in 1988 (published in 1989) as well as his evolving ideas on the topic are published in subsequent papers and chapters—they are worth reading (Lyon, 1989, 1992, 1997b; Lyon, et al., 1997).

In the United Kingdom, Sally McVicker and colleagues developed a formal "befriending" program in which volunteers are trained on communication strategies as well as other needed skills. Then the trained volunteers visit PWA who have recently acquired aphasia in hospitals or in their homes (McVicker, Parr, Pound, & Duchan, 2009). This program is similar in many ways to laryngectomy hospital visitation programs.

Aphasia Conferences

Over the years, there have been a variety of regional aphasia conferences or "Aphasia Days" that are sponsored by hospitals, universities, or Aphasia Centers. When people with aphasia, family members, and friends attend these conferences, they have an opportunity to meet one another during regularly scheduled sessions and/or informally. It's common for people to exchange contact information at these conferences and continue to connect with the people they have met there once they return home.

Aphasia Camps and Cruises

There are a variety of camps offered for PWA and their family members in different regions of North America and beyond. Most operate for a weekend or a week in order to provide aphasia specific programming as well as a variety of recreational opportunities. Similarly, there are a growing number of organizations that are creating "aphasia cruises" by organizing a group of people with aphasia and their family members or friends to sign-up for a specific cruise date. Typically, aphasia specific programming is offered during cruising days at sea with some support provided for negotiating the variety of other cruise activities and port options.

Informal Meetings with Past Clients

Another possibility for SLPs is to think about ways of connecting your present and past clients who are living with aphasia.

Depending on your practice setting, you may be able to invite past clients to your service delivery sites so that people who have more recent aphasia (or have never met others with aphasia) could connect. Before setting up this type of program, you would want to give thought to what type of training or support you would need to provide to a past client who will now be functioning in a new "volunteer" capacity.

Connecting People with Aphasia Online

There are a growing number of Facebook groups that enable people with aphasia, family members, and friends to connect with others who are coping with aphasia. Aphasia Recovery Connection (ARC) manages several Facebook groups including a general group and another specific to care partners of PWA. In addition to the ARC groups, there are also a variety of other Facebook groups available. Although online groups may seem like a perfect solution, we have found that online communication can be quite challenging for some PWA due to the technology and language demands of getting online and navigating software options (Elman, 2001; Elman & Larsen, 2010). Some PWA may need ongoing support and assistance from family members, volunteers, or therapists to access online options.

A: Augmentative & Alternative Communication (AAC)

Why wasn't I provided with another option for communication?

Lynn came to the ACC about six months after her stroke. She had severe apraxia of speech and a mild Broca's aphasia with auditory comprehension more than adequate for conversational speech. Her ability to read was also good. Prior individual therapy had focused on apraxia of speech drills. When Lynn first arrived, she struggled to participate in the aphasia group because it took her such a long time to produce words due to articulatory struggle and her multiple attempts at target word production. She didn't spontaneously employ other strategies in order to assist her communication; however, it became clear to the SLP that with very little clinician prompting and by watching other group members, Lynn began using a combination of writing, gestures, communicative drawing, and various functions on her smart phone to augment her spoken attempts. Her success bred more success. And before long, Lynn was one of the most effective communicators in the group.

When someone has a stroke with motor impairment, physical therapy and occupational therapy are typically provided. As part of his/her evaluation, the physical therapist assesses a variety of equipment that will be used to support the stroke survivor's mobility. Depending on the individual's level of impairment, the physical therapist may determine that a wheelchair, a walker, or a quad cane might be the best support for enabling the person to walk at that point in time. Perhaps a brace or ankle-foot orthosis (AFO) may be needed for additional support. This equipment is provided to enable mobility at that point in time. In addition, therapy is targeted at returning more normal walking through a treatment plan consisting of specific exercises and modalities to assist the return of lower extremity function.

The occupational therapist has a similar goal. She or he evaluates the stroke survivor's ability to perform activities of daily living (ADLs) for such things as bathing, dressing, cooking, shopping, and so forth. Depending on the individual's level of impairment, the occupational therapist may provide equipment such as a grab bar, a bath bench, a bedside commode, a button hook, or a rocking knife to support the individual's ability to perform ADLs at that point in time. In addition, therapy is targeted at returning underlying strength and coordination and a treatment plan is created consisting of specific exercises and activities that will assist the recovery of upper extremity and cognitive functioning for completion of these tasks.

Why aren't SLPs always doing something parallel to this in their assessment and treatment of communicative functioning? Every PWA needs at least one way to communicate! As SLPs, we need to provide effective *communication ramps* to support the exchange of information and enable social interaction. Our assessments need to determine the appropriate supports, at that point in time, that will help make communication easier and more effective for each individual with aphasia.

First of all, you need to find out what is important for that particular person to communicate. Once you know that, you can begin to create communication materials and props that are motivating and useful. Given the pressure for productivity and decreasing time available for formal assessment, you can augment your standardized testing time with some additional data collection methods:

- Gather information using questionnaires about the individual's background and interests that can be completed by family or friends.
- Use activity card sorting options to provides information on specific activities of interest (Haley, Womack, Helm-Estabrooks, Lovette, & Goff, 2013).
- Use social network inventories to learn more about family members and friends (Blackstone & Hunt Berg, 2012; Hilari & Northcott, 2006; Northcott & Hilari, 2011; Northcott, Marshall, & Hilari, 2016; Northcott, Moss, Harrison, & Hilari, 2016; Vickers, 2010).

We live in a "high-tech" society, but I have found that low-tech options are typically best for supporting communication for PWA, especially in the first few months of recovery. Of course there are exceptions to this. But for most PWA, adding a layer of technology to significant communication challenges can result in people becoming less independent. This is because if they aren't independent with using the technology, then they need to look to family members or therapists for assistance with the device. Instead, I consider a variety of low-tech options including the following:

- Developing an individualized communication book and supports.
- Developing a family tree with photos and names of family members, The number of people included can be reduced depending on the needs and abilities of the PWA.
- Using a talking photo book.
- Modeling and encouraging the use of felt tip pens and a pad of paper for writing and drawing.
- Teaching the best yes/no response (head nodding or shaking, pointing, grabbing yes/no knobs, etc.).

- Encouraging and teaching pantomiming and/or specific gestures.
- Using communicative drawing (Lyon, 1995).
- Encouraging writing of words or parts of words.
- Having laminated props such as number lines, scales, maps (local, state, national, world), calendars, cards with numbers, photos of meal choices, and so forth, that are available to support communication and encouraging independent use by PWA (Bernstein-Ellis & Elman, 2007).
- Developing an individualized business card holder system (available in office supply stores) that can hold important individual and business names/addresses. Artifacts can also be inserted such as movie stubs, programs, or receipts to support communication on that topic in the future.

In their text, Simmons-Mackie, King, and Beukelman (2013) provide additional examples of using communication supports at all levels on the continuum of care. SLPs may also find the Famous People Protocol (2019) useful for uncovering communicative strengths and strategies, especially for those living with severe aphasia (Holland, Forbes, Fromm, & MacWhinney, 2019).

P: Partner Training

Why didn't someone show me how to have a conversation with my spouse?

One of the services we provide at the ACC is a "second opinion" evaluation. I had received a call from a wife, Deb, who asked if she could schedule a second opinion evaluation with me for her husband, Dean. She explained that he had received 18 months of individual therapy since his stroke, but he still had severe aphasia and she wondered if there was anything else they could do. I asked her to send me copies of his speech-language pathology notes and reports, so I could determine what the SLP had worked on since his stroke. The notes indicated that treatment had focused on apraxia of speech drills with some general language stimulation. When Dean and Deb arrived, I began the session by gathering some biographical information from both of them and then asked Deb to wait outside during my aphasia test and diagnostic probe administration. The testing revealed that Dean had a moderate apraxia of speech, a mild dysarthria, and a moderate mixed aphasia. Dean also displayed some emotional lability and I noted some challenges with secretion management. I invited Deb back into the room so we could continue our discussion about what each of their future communication and life goals were. On the table in front of us were some local, state, national, and world maps, a number line, and a calendar. We each had a pad of paper and a felt tip pen. I had "discovered" during my diagnostic probes with Dean, a set of possible communication tools and strategies to support his conversation. Before long, with some support and guidance provided by me, Dean was indicating that his goals were the following: to travel to Europe (he used the world map to point to the specific countries); to spend time at their vacation home in Southern California the following month (he used the state map and the calendar); and to go wine tasting in Napa Valley (he pointed to the map and drew a wine glass). Deb reminded him that her father was quite ill and she didn't feel as though she could leave the country for a vacation. And she told me that she was afraid that if he took a break from therapy, that he would lose ground, and that the loss would be permanent. I realized right then that neither one had taken a single day off in the 18 months since his stroke. I reassured Deb that participating in activities that interested both of them was exactly what they should be doing. And the next time I looked up, Deb was crying. When I asked her why, she told me, "Why didn't anyone else ever show me how to have a conversation with Dean?"

The importance of a well-trained communication partner cannot be overestimated for people living with moderate-to-severe aphasia. A trained partner becomes a vital communication ramp for successful use of the communicative supports and strategies that are identified by the SLP. Clinicians and researchers have taken several different approaches when training partners of PWA. Beyond the scope of the current chapter, a systematic review of the communication partner literature is available in Simmons-Mackie, Raymer, Armstrong, Holland, and Cherney (2010) and updated in Simmons-Mackie, Raymer, and Cherney (2016). I'd like to share several communication partner approaches in this chapter. All of the approaches have the SLP working with the dyad (PWA and partner) as a unit.

Alarcon, Hickey, Rogers, and Olswang (1997) start with videotaping family members and the PWA communicating. The SLP then provides structured viewing for the dyad, giving specific feedback of both the successful and unsuccessful interactions. Lyon (1996, 1997a) provides intervention to the dyad through review of pre- and poststroke activities with each member of the dyad selecting activities that they want to resume. The SLP then provides counseling and training to encourage resumption of these activities. Boles and Lewis (2003) discuss solution-focused aphasia therapy in which a SLP and social worker work together with the dyad to help find effective strategies and solutions for issues that they identify.

The partner training approach that has received the most research and replication is Supported Conversation for Aphasia™ (SCA™). This training was developed by Aura Kagan and her colleagues at the Aphasia Institute in Toronto. SCA™ training concentrates on methods of acknowledging and revealing the communicative competence of PWA. Acknowledging competence includes ways of making sure that the PWA is being treated respectfully. Revealing competence includes the strategies and methods that the PWA and partner learn to use for giving and receiving information needed for successful communication. Figure 2–2 provides the variety of communication modalities or "tools" that are available to PWA and partners. During instruction, the PWA and partner receive training in those communicative tools that are most likely to be successful in order to get information "In" (listening and reading) and "Out" (speaking and writing). The dyad also learns methods to "Verify" that accurate information has been shared.

The Aphasia Institute provides SCA™ training in Toronto but has also made available a variety of online resources on their

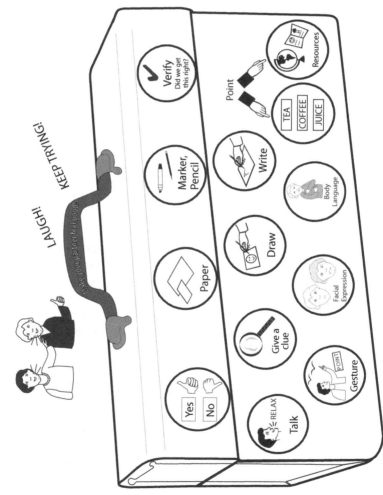

Figure 2–2. Communication toolbox. © 2012, Aphasia Institute. Reprinted with permission of Aphasia Institute.

website at no cost. I frequently refer appropriate family members to their online training module entitled, "An Introduction to Supported Conversation for Adults with Aphasia (SCA™) Self-Directed Learning Module" (Aphasia Institute, n.d.). SLPs that are not familiar with SCA™ will also find this module extremely helpful!

E: Education & Resources

Why didn't anyone ever explain aphasia to me in a way I could understand?

> I try to accept as many invitations as I can to talk about aphasia and communication strategies with local community stroke groups. I make sure that my presentations are "aphasia friendly" by presenting information at a slower rate of speech, using simplified vocabulary, and including PowerPoint slides that enable me to combine photographs, pictographs, written key words, and other graphics along with my spoken presentation. I also like to include videoclips. Following one of my presentations, Rebecca raised her hand to ask me a question. She was a stroke survivor with aphasia following a hemorrhagic stroke that had been caused by an aneurysm. She was attending my presentation with her husband and it seemed as though it was the first time she had been in a room with others who had aphasia. Rebecca explained that it had been about two years since her stroke. She wanted to let me know that my presentation had helped her understand a lot about her own aphasia for the first time. Then she asked, "Why didn't anyone ever explain aphasia to me in a way I could understand?"

People who are living with aphasia are at an extreme disadvantage when it comes to finding out about the disorder itself. How would you typically learn about a medical disorder that you have? Many of us would get online and "google" the name of the disorder to learn more. Or we might talk to friends or family members who have the disorder. Or we might read a book or an article that includes information about treatment options "and prognosis. However, these methods may be very challenging for someone living with aphasia, as the language barrier caused by the disorder itself can make reading or conversation difficult, or for some, impossible. Instead, PWA need to receive information in an "aphasia friendly" format. An aphasia friendly format should not only be used for information about aphasia itself, but also when sharing any information that would typically be given verbally (spoken or written). This means that sharing information about all transactional needs should be made aphasia friendly for the PWA including receiving information about medical procedures and informed consent, community resources, financial and banking requirements, and so forth. Aphasia friendly techniques include use of pictographs to augment text, simplifying grammar and vocabulary of words used, slowing rate of speech, reducing distractions, such as environmental noise or visual distractors, and using additional "white space" to reduce visual complexity. Each PWA will have his/her own preferences for those techniques and strategies that assist in accessing spoken and written information more successfully. One of the roles of the SLP is to share information about aphasia-friendly techniques and strategies with other professionals, organizations, and businesses so that they can create appropriate materials. At the Aphasia Center of California, we decided to include aphasia-friendly summary webpages for all of the sections on our website. Accessed via an "Aphasia Friendly" button near the top of the page, the content and format of these pages is simplified and pictographs are paired with the text (http://www.aphasiacenter.org).

Family members and friends also need information about aphasia. We know from the aphasia awareness literature that they are unlikely to be familiar with the disorder (Elman, Ogar, & Elman, 2000; Simmons-Mackie, 2018). We also know from the research literature that many family members and friends report that they did not receive adequate information about aphasia from health care professionals (Avent et al., 2005; Brown et al., 2012; Elman et al., 2016; Hilton et al., 2014; Hinckley et al., 2013; Howe et al., 2012; Wallace et al., 2017; Worrall, et al., 2011). SLPs may want to create a handout for families that includes some basic information about aphasia; a listing of websites and community resources where they can learn more and get support from other family member; titles of firsthand accounts in books and articles about aphasia; names and contact information for local aphasia programs; and so forth. I believe that it is never too early in the recovery process to provide this information. Even if the family member isn't ready to read further at the point of time you are working with them, my experience has been that they may read your handout later, when they may have more time and interest.

Some Closing Thoughts

Life participation and the social imperative are focused on reestablishing meaningful skills and desired activities as well as desired social contacts. Speech-language pathologists must focus on using the perspective of the PWA and family members in order to optimize communication skills and improve quality of life. And I hope that using the C.A.P.E. checklist and categories will help you to prioritize your intervention, especially in the early months of recovery. You have the opportunity to make a real difference in the lives of people living with aphasia!

I have been working at the ACC for nearly 25 years. There have been times that I have felt overwhelmed and frustrated. But, in all this time, I have never once felt the same sense of clinical failure that I did years ago. Sometimes, clinical successes have been more challenging than others. But I am certain that the PWA, family members, and friends, who have shared their lives with us while participating in ACC programs, are now living more successfully because of the community that we've built together. I'll end this chapter with my very favorite quote, by the anthropologist Margaret Mead: "Never doubt that a small group of committed people can change the world; indeed, it is the only thing that ever has."

References

Alarcon, N., Hickey, E., Rogers, M., & Olswang, L. (1997, March). *Family based intervention for chronic aphasia*. Paper presented at the Nontraditional Approaches to Aphasia Conference, Yountville, CA.

Aphasia Institute. (n.d.). *Life participation approach to aphasia: A statement of values for the future.* This version of the article includes LPAA examples and the full reference list. Retrieved from https://www.aphasia.ca/wp-content/uploads/2011/01/LPAA_AI.pdf

Aphasia Institute. (n.d.). *An introduction to Supported Conversation for Adults with Aphasia (SCA™) self-directed learning module.* Retrieved from http://www.aphasia.ca/

Aphasia Institute. (2012). *Toolbox.* Retrieved from Aphasia Institute Training Materials on Supported Conversation for Adults with Aphasia (SCA™).

Aphasia United Best Practice Statements. (n.d.). Retrieved from Aphasia United website http://www.aphasiaunited.org/

Attard, M., Lanyon, L., Togher, L., & Rose, M. (2015). Consumer perspectives on community aphasia groups: A narrative literature review in the context of psychological well-being. *Aphasiology, 29*(8), 983–1019.

Aten, J., Caliguri, M., & Holland, A. (1982). The efficacy of functional communication therapy for chronic aphasic patients. *Journal of Speech and Hearing Disorders, 47*, 93–96.

Avent, J., Glista, S., Wallace, S., Jackson, J., Nishioka, J., & Yip, W. (2005). Family information needs about aphasia. *Aphasiology, 19*(3–5), 365–375.

Bernstein-Ellis, E., & Elman, R. (2006). *The Book Connection™: A life participation book club for individuals with acquired reading impairment.* Oakland, CA: Aphasia Center of California. http://www.aphasiacenter.org

Bernstein-Ellis, E., & Elman, R. (2007). Group communication treatment for individuals with aphasia: The Aphasia Center of California approach. In R. Elman (Ed.), *Group treatment for neurogenic communication disorders: The expert clinician's approach* (2nd ed.). San Diego, CA: Plural Publishing.

Blackstone, S. W., & Hunt Berg, M. (2012). *Social networks: A communication inventory for individuals with complex communication needs and their communication partners.* Monterey, CA: ACI.

Boles, L., & Lewis, M. (2003). Working with couples: Solution focused aphasia therapy. *Asia Pacific Journal of Speech, Language and Hearing, 8*(3), 153–159.

Bollinger, R., Musson, N., & Holland, A. (1993). A study of group communication intervention with chronically aphasic persons. *Aphasiology, 7*, 301–313.

Brown, K., Worrall, L. E., Davidson, B., & Howe, T. (2012). Living successfully with aphasia: A qualitative meta-analysis of the perspectives of individuals with aphasia, family members, and speech-language pathologists. *International Journal of Speech-Language Pathology, 14*(2), 141–155.

Elman, R. J. (2001). The Internet and aphasia: Crossing the digital divide. *Aphasiology, 15*(10/11), 895–899.

Elman, R. J. (Ed.). (2007a). *Group treatment of neurogenic communication disorders: The expert clinician's approach* (2nd ed.). San Diego, CA: Plural Publishing.

Elman, R. J. (2007b). The importance of aphasia group treatment for rebuilding community and health. *Topics in Language Disorders, 27*(4), 300–308.

Elman, R. J. (2011, 2018c). Social and life participation approaches to aphasia intervention. In L. LaPointe (Ed.), *Aphasia and related neurogenic language disorders* (5th ed). New York, NY: Thieme Medical.

Elman, R. J. (2013, November). *CAPE: Making choices in aphasia intervention when intensive therapy is not possible.* Presented to the ASHA Convention, Chicago, IL.

Elman, R. J. (2016). Aphasia centers and the life participation approach to aphasia: A paradigm shift. *Topics in Language Disorders, 36*(2), 154–167.

Elman, R. J. (2018a, December). *Conversation groups for people with aphasia: Rationale and evidence.* [Video webinar]. Seattle, WA: MedBridge. Retrieved from https://www.medbridgeeducation.com/courses/details/conversation-groups-for-people-with-aphasia-ratio nale-and-evidence-roberta-elman-speech-language-pathology-aphasia

Elman, R. J. (2018b, December). *Conversation groups for people with aphasia: Techniques and application.* [Video webinar]. Seattle, WA: MedBridge. Retrieved from https://www.medbridgeeducation.com/courses/details/conversation-groups-for-people-with-aphasia-tech niques-and-application-roberta-elman-speech-language-pathology-aphasia

Elman, R. J. (2020). Ethical responsibilities to adults with communication impairments involved in group therapy. *Seminars in Speech and Language, 41*(3), 241–248.

Elman, R. J., & Bernstein-Ellis, E. (1999a). The efficacy of group communication treatment in adults with chronic aphasia. *Journal of Speech, Language, and Hearing Research, 42,* 411–419.

Elman, R. J., & Bernstein-Ellis, E. (1999b). Psychosocial aspects of group communication treatment: Preliminary findings. *Seminars in Speech & Language, 20*(1) 65–72.

Elman, R. J., Cohen, A., & Silverman, M. (2016, May). *Perceptions of speech-language pathology services provided to person with aphasia: A caregiver survey.* Presented to the Clinical Aphasiology Conference, Charlottesville, VA.

Elman, R. J., & Larson, S. (2010, May). *Computer and internet use among people with aphasia.* Paper presented to the Clinical Aphasiology Conference, Isle of Palms, SC.

Elman, R. J., Ogar, J., & Elman, S. (2000). Aphasia: Awareness, advocacy, and activism. *Aphasiology, 14*(5/6), 455–459.

Ewing, S. (2007). Group process, group dynamics, and group techniques with neurogenic communication disorders. In R. Elman (Ed.), *Group treatment for neurogenic communication disorders: The expert clinician's approach* (2nd ed.). San Diego, CA: Plural Publishing.

Haley, K., Womack, J., Helm-Estabrooks, N., Lovette, B., & Goff, R. (2013). Supporting autonomy for people with aphasia: Use of the Life Interests and Values (LIV) cards. *Topics in Stroke Rehabilitation, 20*(1), 22–35.

Hilari, K., & Northcott, S. (2006). Social support in people with chronic aphasia. *Aphasiology, 20*(1), 17–36.

Hilton, R., Leenhouts, S., Webster, J., & Morris, J. (2014). Information, support and training needs of relatives of people with aphasia: Evidence from the literature. *Aphasiology, 28*(7), 797–822.

Hinckley, J. J., Hasselkus, A., & Ganzfried, E. (2013). What people living with aphasia think about the availability of aphasia resources. *American Journal of Speech-Language Pathology, 22*(2), S310–S317.

Holland, A., Forbes, M., Fromm, D., & MacWhinney, B. (2019). Communicative strengths in severe aphasia: The famous people protocol and its value in planning treatment. *American Journal of Speech-Language Pathology, 28*(3), 1010–1018.

Howe, R., Davidson, B., Worrall, L., Hersh, D., Ferguson, A., Sherratt, S., & Gilbert, J. (2012). You need to rehab . . . families as well: Family members' own goals for aphasia rehabilitation. *International Journal of Language and Communication Disorders, 47*, 522–521.

Kagan, A. (1998). Supported conversation for adults with aphasia: Methods and resources for training conversation partners. *Aphasiology, 12*(9), 816–830.

Kagan, A., Black, S., Duchan, J., Simmons-Mackie, N., & Square, P. (2001). Training volunteers as conversation partners using "Supported Conversations for Adults with Aphasia" (SCA): A controlled trial. *Journal of Speech, Language, and Hearing Research, 44*(3), 624–638.

Kagan, A., Simmons-Mackie, N., Rowland, A., Huijbregts, M., Shumway, E., McEwen, W., . . . Sharp, S. (2007). Counting what counts: A framework for capturing real-life outcomes of aphasia intervention. *Aphasiology, 22*(3), 258–280.

Kearns, K., & Elman, R. (2001, 2008). Group therapy for aphasia: Theoretical and practical considerations. In R. Chapey (Ed.), *Language intervention strategies in aphasia and related neurogenic communication disorders* (5th ed., pp. 316–337). Baltimore, MD: Lippincott, Williams & Wilkins.

Lanyon, L., Rose, M., & Worrall, L. (2013). The efficacy of outpatient and community-based aphasia group interventions: A systematic review. *International Journal of Speech-Language Pathology, 15*(4), 359–374.

LPAA Project Group (Chapey, R., Duchan, J., Elman, R., Garcia, L., Kagan, A., Lyon, J., & Simmons-Mackie, N.) (2000). Life participation approach to aphasia: A statement of values for the future. *ASHA Leader, 5*(3), 4–6. Retrieved from https://leader.pubs.asha.org/doi/10.1044/leader.FTR.05032000.4 Reprinted in R. Chapey (2001/2008) (Ed.). *Language intervention strategies in aphasia and related neurogenic communication disorders* (5th ed.). Baltimore, MD: Lippincott, Williams & Wilkins.

Lyon, J. (1989). Communication partners: Their value in reestablishing communication with aphasic adults. In T. Prescott (Ed.), *Clinical aphasiology conference proceedings* (Vol. 18, pp. 11–17). Boston, MA: College-Hill.

Lyon, J. (1992). Communicative use and participation in life for aphasic adults in natural settings: The scope of the problem. *American Journal of Speech and Language Pathology, 1*(3), 7–14.

Lyon, J. (1995). Drawing: Its value as a communication aid for adults with aphasia. *Aphasiology, 9*(1), 33–94.

Lyon, J. (1996). Optimizing communication and participation in life for aphasic adults and their prime caregivers in natural settings: A use model for treatment. In G. Wallace (Ed.), *Adult aphasia rehabilitation* (pp. 137–160). Newton, MA: Butterworth Heinemann.

Lyon, J. (1997a). Treating real-life functionality in a couple coping with severe aphasia. In N. Helm-Estabrooks & A. Holland (Eds.), *Approaches to the treatment of aphasia* (pp. 203–239). San Diego, CA: Singular Publishing.

Lyon, J. (1997b). Volunteers and partners: Moving intervention outside the treatment room. In B. Shadden & M. Toner (Eds.), *Communication and aging* (pp. 299–324). Austin, TX: Pro-Ed.

Lyon, J., Cariski, D., Keisler, L., Rosenbek, J., Levine, R., & Kumpula, J. (1997). Communication partners: Enhancing participation in life and communication for adults with aphasia in natural settings. *Aphasiology, 11*, 693–708.

McVicker S., Parr S., Pound, C., & Duchan J. (2009). The communication partner scheme: A project to develop long-term, low-cost access to conversation for people living with aphasia. *Aphasiology, 23*(1), 52–71.

Northcott, S., & Hilari, K. (2011). Why do people lose their friends after a stroke? *International Journal of Language & Communication Disorders, 46*(5), 524–534.

Northcott, S., Marshall, J., & Hilari, K. (2016). What factors predict who will have a strong social network following a stroke? *Journal of Speech, Language, and Hearing Research, 59,* 772–783.

Northcott, S., Moss, B., Harrison, K., & Hilari, K. (2016). A systematic review of the impact of stroke on social support and social networks: Associated factors and patterns of change. *Clinical Rehabilitation, 38*(8), 811–831.

Parr, S., Byng, S., Gilpin, S., & Ireland, S. (1997). *Talking about aphasia: Living with loss of language after stroke.* Buckingham, UK: Open University Press.

Pound, C., Parr, S., Lindsay, J., & Woolf, C. (2000). *Beyond aphasia: Therapies for living with communication disability.* Oxon, UK: Winslow Press.

Power, E., Thomas, E., Worrall, L, Rose, M., Togher, L, Nickels, L., . . . Clarke, K. (2015). Development and validation of Australian aphasia rehabilitation best practice statements using the RAND/UCLA appropriateness method. *BMJ Open, 5,* e007641.

Rose, M. L., & Attard, M. C. (2015). Practices and challenges in community aphasia groups in Australia: Results of a national survey. *International Journal of Speech-Language Pathology, 17,* 241–251.

Simmons-Mackie, N. (2018). *Aphasia in North America.* Moorestown, NJ: Aphasia Access.

Simmons-Mackie, N., King, J. M., & Beukelman, D. R. (Eds.). (2013). *Supporting communication for adults with acute and chronic aphasia.* Towson, MD: Brookes.

Simmons-Mackie, N., Raymer, A., Armstrong, E., Holland, A., & Cherney, L. (2010). Communication partner training in aphasia: A systematic review. *Archives of Physical Medicine and Rehabilitation, 91*(12), 1814–1837.

Simmons-Mackie, N., Raymer, A., & Cherney, L. R. (2016). Communication partner training in aphasia: An updated systematic review. *Archives of Physical Medicine and Rehabilitation, 97*(12), 2202–2221.

Thompson, C. K., Shapiro, L. P., Kiran, S., & Sobecks, J. (2003). The role of syntactic complexity in treatment of sentence deficits in agrammatic aphasia. *Journal of Speech, Language, and Hearing Research, 46*(3), 591–607.

Van der Gaag, A., Smith, L., Davies, S., Moss, B., Cornelius, V., Laing, S., & Mowles, C. (2005).Therapy and support services for people with long term stroke and aphasia and their relatives: A six month follow up study. *Clinical Rehabilitation, 19,* 372–381.

Vickers, C. P. (2010). Social networks after the onset of aphasia: The impact of aphasia group attendance. *Aphasiology, 24*(6–8), 902–913.

Wallace, S. J., Worrall, L., Rose, T., Le Dorze, G., Cruice, M., Isaksen, J., . . . Gauvreau, C. A. (2017). Which outcomes are most important to people with aphasia and their families? An international nominal group technique study framed within the ICF. *Disability & Rehabilitation, 39,* 1364–1379.

Wertz, R., Collins, M., Weiss, D., Kurtzke, J., Friden, R., Brookshire, R., . . . Resurreccion, E. (1981). Veterans administration cooperative study on aphasia: A comparison of individual and group treatment. *Journal of Speech and Hearing Research, 24,* 580–594.

Worrall, L., Sherratt, S., Rogers, P., Howe, T., Hersh, D., Ferguson, A., & Davidson, R. (2011). What people with aphasia want: Their goals according to the ICF. *Aphasiology, 25,* 309–322.

World Health Organization. (2001). *International classification of functioning, disability and health, ICF.* Geneva, Switzerland: Author.

DISCOVERING FUNCTIONAL NEEDS IN SPEECH-LANGUAGE THERAPY

Sarah Baar

Introduction

Imagine a dream scenario: A client comes to the speech-language pathology assessment and within minutes, the speech-language pathologist (SLP) knows that he wants help speaking in order to have more meaningful conversations with his friends about golf, and he also wants help with his memory in order to better check and record his daily blood sugar.

Does this situation sound familiar? Most likely, it's a rare scenario in the work settings of most speech-language pathologists.

Eliciting functional needs tends to be elusive. In fact, one of the most challenging needs within our field concerns how to provide speech-language therapy through a Life Participation approach (LPAA Project Group, 2000). The problem is not the willingness of the SLPs. Given the scenario above, an SLP would jump at the chance to use speech-language therapy as a vehicle to improve those specific life needs. The true challenge in providing speech-language therapy with a Life Participation approach is how to discover and meet functional needs **within the constraints of your work setting**.

Discovering functional needs during an assessment is difficult for many reasons: Productivity demands lead to workflow decisions that include workbook activities and depersonalization of tasks. Clients and coworkers are unfamiliar with how an SLP can assist with meeting functional needs, because our traditional, impairment-focused approach leans away from explicitly describing how we can impact real life activities. Insurance requirements and reimbursement policies may emphasize a focus on standardized testing results alone, leaving less time to discover functional needs. Shorter lengths-of-stay in acute or rehabilitation settings may discourage SLPs from starting to address life participation. Finally, speech-language therapy materials that have historically been in the "therapy closet" don't inherently link to real life needs.

Discrepancies exist between what the client views as being relevant and what the SLP views as relevant. Chart reviews have indicated SLPs say they value participation, but it doesn't match up with what they are actually doing in therapy (Torrence, Baylor, Yorkston, & Spencer, 2016). A participation approach is quite different from the traditional "impairment-focused" model, and so SLPs aren't necessarily providing better person-centered care as they become more experienced (Dilollo & Favreau, 2010). These various constraints play out in different ways in different settings, but ultimately some of these factors impact almost every SLP in a traditional medical setting.

In the midst of growing demands and changes in these medical settings, our own speech-language pathology research has also grown—exploded—showing the value of focusing on meaningful, personally-relevant goals and treatment for each patient (Davenport, Dickson, & Minns Lowe, 2019; Worrall, 2019; Wray, Clarke, & Forster, 2019). Our own field has adopted the World Health Organization's International Classification Framework (WHO-ICF, 2001). Rather than focusing only on impairment, the ICF framework emphasizes the whole person and how someone's activity and participation is impacted following the onset of cognitive-communication disorders. With the implementation of the Affordable Care Act in 2011, a person-centered approach has blossomed as the standard for all health care. Why is this? Research has shown that a person-centered approach to health care leads to better, more efficient outcomes, and with greater patient satisfaction. (Epstein, Fiscella, Lesser, & Strange, 2010). Patients themselves have also told us that in order to stay relevant and helpful as a profession, we need to focus treatment on activities that are meaningful to them (Yorkston, Baylor, & Britton, 2017; Worrall et al., 2011).

Here lies the crux of the issue: we may know that research supports using a personalized approach that focuses on life participation. And yet, with the myriad of constraints listed above that are the reality in various medical settings, it is not clear how to proceed. In fact, it's often thought that the Life Participation approach can be used "down the road" when the acute phase of recovery is done, and when a university clinic, or groups, or aphasia centers can take over and treat outside of a traditional insurance model.

And so, in the climate of increasing pressure and constraints for the medical SLP, the question becomes: How do we do this? How do we discover functional needs when we have less time than ever? What tools can we use that are both supported by evidence and quick in a busy work setting? Are we in need of therapy material shift, or a mind shift? Although the ever-changing health care climate may be hard to face for the bravest of clinicians, it offers us freedom to look at how we spend our therapy time in a fresh light. It is at this intersection that the Life Participation approach mindset can begin.

My aim for this chapter is to provide the everyday clinical SLP with ideas, tools, and tips for how to use what we know is best practice: A person-centered approach from the assessment forward—and to fit this approach within the constraints that may be present in various medical settings.

A Mindset Shift

The first tool for discovering and meeting functional needs may be a mindset shift for the SLP. The mindset shift begins with our understanding that a Life Participation approach will broaden how we view the goals we can meet in speech-language therapy. The Life Participation approach uses a holistic framework to conceptualize all the ways someone's overall functioning and quality of life can be impacted. These factors are divided into domains that overlap and affect one another (Figure 3–1). Kagan and Simmons-Mackie (2007) describe these as:

- Personal Factors/Identity
- Impairment (e.g., Aphasia)
- Environment
- Participation

Because our traditional focus was on the impairment only, our goals and treatment plans reflected work in that domain alone. With the more holistic framework, our goals and treatments can clearly expand to working within any of the domains listed, as they all affect one another.

To use a nonclinical example that shows the benefit of broadening our mindset to a holistic view of participation, let's imagine a friend who takes up running as a hobby. When you ask your friend how running is going, consider all the different responses your friend could give that would indicate a successful answer:

- Personal Factors/Identity: "I am loving it! It's really made me appreciate how strong my body is. I never thought I could do this, but it's made me feel so confident about what I can do."
- Impairment: "I cut 3 minutes off my last 5K! I'm getting faster."

Framework for Outcome Measurement (FROM)

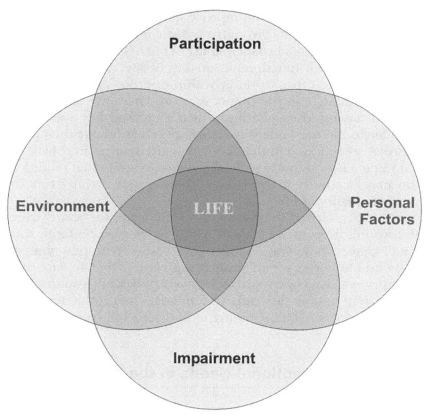

Figure 3–1. FROM domains (Kagan et al., 2008). © 2008 Aphasia Institute. Reprinted with permission from Aphasia Institute.

- ■ Environment: "It's going better. When I started, I was running on trails that were giving me knee injuries, but I figured it out. So now I'm picking paved trails and I haven't had any injuries since I switched."
- ■ Participation: "It has been such a nice outlet for me. I've joined a local running group and we meet up 3×/ week. It's given me something to look forward to each week."

In this example, any of these answers could be considered a success! The friend does not necessarily have to improve running time for this new hobby to improve quality of life. Can you see how viewing situations through a holistic framework allows you to take into account a broadened list of factors that may improve someone's overall functioning, quality of life, and confidence? You can also see that working within one domain may impact another domain (e.g., the runner improved her environment and stopped having knee injuries, which increased her speed and confidence.) In the same way, using speech-language therapy to improve someone's confidence with participating in a task, or making it easier to participate through environmental modification may be the best use of speech-language therapy time to improve quality of life!

This broadened mindset will set the stage for you to view discovering functional needs in a holistic, person-centered way. It will change how you conduct your assessment, how you set goals, and how you spend your therapy time. The Life Participation approach isn't one tool to selectively pull out of your toolbox for the right patient; instead, it's a mindset that influences your therapy process from beginning to end for each patient.

Discovering Functional Needs in the Assessment

When adopting the Life Participation approach mindset, it becomes important to efficiently discover functional needs in the assessment visit. The following tools may be used in various combinations to assist with discovering functional needs.

Nonstandardized Assessment

We will first discuss tools that fall under the umbrella of the nonstandardized portion of the assessment. The nonstandardized assessment is where tasks or tools will give more in-depth information about someone's needs, how activity/participation may be affected, and what context/environment they may be functioning in. It also gives information about family support or communication partners.

Nonstandardized assessment is increasingly important. As research has shown, there is a lack of correlation between impairment-level results and someone's activity and participation (Coelho, Ylvisaker & Turkstra, 2005; LeBlanc, Hayden & Paulman, 2000; Whyte & Barrett, 2013). This means that in order to understand someone's everyday functioning, we need more information than a standardized test score alone. If someone has mild-moderate memory challenges by testing, will they be able to take care of a pet? Can they still manage to cook meals for themselves? Are they able to do their job tasks? In order to gain a full picture of someone's functioning, nonstandardized assessment is vital.

Using nonstandardized assessment procedures is not a new notion—in fact, it is recommended as a best practice for Aphasia, Primary Progressive Aphasia (PPA), Traumatic Brain Injury (TBI), Motor Speech Disorders, Dementia, Autism, and beyond (American Speech-Language-Hearing Association Practice Portal, n.d.). There are several different tools that can be used solely or in different combinations with one another, with the primary goal of discovering functional needs.

Motivational Interviewing

How we choose to phrase our words in speech-language therapy can make a difference in motivating our clients to participate and engage in the therapy process. Motivational Interviewing is a person-centered interaction style, and evidence-based for supporting change and supporting goal setting and motivation for therapy (MacFarlane, 2012). Using Motivational Interviewing techniques throughout the assessment can establish a cooperative and change-focused relationship from the first visit. Motivational Interviewing emphasizes four key principles that should be kept in mind throughout interactions with the client:

- Express Empathy
- Develop Discrepancy
- Roll with Resistance
- Support Self-Efficacy

In addition to supporting these four principles, Motivational Interviewing uses the following interaction styles selectively to focus the conversation upon change and help lead the patient down that road.

- Open Questions/Statements: Questions and statements are phrased in an open-ended manner, so that the client is allowed to take the response in the direction that is important to them. Closed, yes/no questions are avoided.
- Affirmations: Affirmations are statements that highlight strengths and facts in a way that differs from a compliment. This technique allows the SLP to recognize the client's skills or appreciate them in a genuine way.
- Reflections: Reflections are important in letting a client know that you are really listening. These statements can be as simple as rephrasing what the client said, or more complex by adding meaning while rephrasing what the client said. As you start with this skill, use one reflection for each question you ask, and as you get better, use two reflections for each question you ask. Studies have shown that we need to do more of these as speech-language pathologists! (MacFarlane, 2012).
- Summaries: Summarizing is a technique that involves consolidating a discussion. The point of summarizing is to highlight change talk, promote strengths, consolidate information, and move the discussion forward.

For examples of each technique being applied to different parts of the clinical process, see Table 3–1.

Person-Centered Outcomes

Person-Centered Outcomes (PCOs) are questionnaires or surveys that may be completed by the client, speech therapist, or communication partner. Many of them give a broadened view of how certain activities or participation at home may be going, or they may include a broader view of function by looking at confidence or quality of life within life scenarios. These questionnaires are scored, which can be helpful for measuring improvement in participation or confidence, rather than an impairment score.

Table 3–1. Examples of Motivational Interviewing Techniques Applied to the Clinical Process

	Open Questions	Affirmations	Reflections	Summaries
Assessment	What's most important for us to talk about today? What's going well at home? Describe a typical day.	You care so much for your spouse, and you're taking a lot of information into consideration; that can be tricky. Your life has changed a lot and you are keeping a positive attitude.	You are feeling angry that therapy has been recommended by your doctor. It sounds like things aren't going quite the same as normal at home, but you aren't sure if you want to spend time in speech therapy.	Summarize history and then: "What else?" You aren't sure what goals you've had in earlier therapies, but ultimately you want to return home, so you may be willing to participate with the goal of getting back home.
Goal-Setting	What might your life look like if you were at a point that you didn't even need speech therapy?	It sounds like you want to make some changes with your attention at home, and you're confident that you are someone who can make those changes.	You are feeling frustrated about how slow progress has been. You're noticing that you've misplaced your keys or coffee mug, but it's not really bothering you.	You haven't enjoyed the speech therapy tasks you did in inpatient rehab, and you still have goals that you want to improve for how things are going at home before you return to work.
Therapy	Tell me more about what you're noticing. What did you think about that task?	I see you concentrating to do this the best you can.	You are feeling _____ about _____. It sounds like	Today you recognized:
Home Program	What may be a way you could practice this at home?	You are working really hard at the new routine at home.	It sounds like your family has noticed some of the word-finding problems, and it kind of hurts your feelings to realize they've noticed a change.	You considered _____ and started problem-solving by _____, and it worked well for you.

For example, the Communicative Confidence Rating Scale for Aphasia (CCRSA) asks questions about answering the phone, talking with strangers, or understanding conversation in a noisy restaurant (Babbitt & Cherney, 2010). This particular PCO gives information about confidence, not ability. And so, if someone rates themselves poorly on two key areas and agrees they would like to be more confident with those tasks, you have some activity information to incorporate into therapy. Additionally, because the PCOs have a score associated with them, it may be helpful to incorporate the score into goal setting to actually show improved confidence or participation. Here is an example of a goal that targets increasing confidence: "The patient will improve confidence in communication settings as measured by Communicative Confidence Rating Scale for Aphasia (Baseline score xxx)." PCOs continue to gain momentum in our field as we increasingly recognize the value of the person's experience with a cognitive-communication disorder. For a list of PCOs that you can access freely, and the population they are developed for, see Table 3–2.

Setting-Specific Needs Checklist

A setting-specific checklist is essentially a semistructured interview based on what setting the client is in, and what needs they may have within that setting. Because clients may not always be able to determine or express functional needs with an open-ended question (e.g., How could your memory work better?), a semistructured list of common needs in a particular setting may help determine how the SLP can improve the client's function right within that setting (e.g., Are you able to use your TV remote? Have you been successful with keeping track of appointments?) The use of a semistructured interview has been successful in eliciting more needs with clients in a recent study with clients with dementia (Dutzi, Schwenk, Kirchner, Bauer, & Hauer, 2019), and I've found it efficient and meaningful in my own practice with the adult neurogenic population. See Table 3–3 for an example of a Setting-Specific Needs Checklist and Contextual Observation for Inpatient Rehab.

Table 3–2. Person-Centered Outcomes with Free Access

Name of PCO	Designed For:	Where to Find:
CCRSA: Communication Confidence Rating Scale for Aphasia	People with aphasia rate their confidence in participating in various situations	Email lcherney@ sralab.org to request a copy
COAST: Communication Outcome After Stroke	People with communication changes after stroke	Make an account and request permission for free access: https:// www.click2go.umip .com/i/coa/coast.html
CES: Communicative Effectiveness Survey	People with dysarthria (including due to Parkinson's disease)	Open as PDF and Print Appendix: https:// pubs.asha.org/doi/ pdf/10.1044/1058-0360 %282008/07-0010%29
CPIB: Communicative Participation Item Bank	Community-dwelling adults with communication changes due to spasmodic dysphonia, multiple sclerosis, Parkinson's disease, amyotrophic lateral sclerosis, or head and neck cancer	https://www.ncbi.nlm. nih.gov/pmc/articles/ PMC4377222/ Table 2 (Open in a separate window to print)
PCRS: Patient Competency Rating Scale	Client, caregiver, or clinician to evaluate self-awareness after brain injury Includes option to compare multiple perspectives	http://www.tbims.org/ combi/pcrs/pcrsrat.html
The Vocal Priority Questionnaire	People with voice disorders to identify priorities of vocal attributes to target in therapy	Open as PDF and print Appendix C: https://pubs.asha.org/ doi/10.1044/2018_ JSLHR-S-18-0109

Table 3–3. Setting-Specific Needs Checklist and Contextual Observation for Inpatient Rehab

Functional Need	Conversation Prompts/Observation
Use Call Light	Have you been able to use your call light? Show me how you use it.
Medical Diagnosis/ Knowledge	Can you tell me why you are here? What have you learned about your medical condition?
Order Meal	Have you been able to order a meal? Tell me what you would order for dinner.
Phone Call/Text	Have you been able to make a phone call? Show me how you would call someone.
Use Calendar/ Schedule	Are you using a schedule? Show me how you know what is going on for the day.
Follow PT/OT Recommendations	What recommendations have PT/OT give you? How will you remember to do what they recommend?
Find Different Locations Within the Building	Have you been able to find your way around the building? How do you remember your room number?
Communicate Needs to Nursing	Have you been able to tell nursing when you need something? What would you say if you were cold?
Medication Names/ Purposes	Are you on some new medications? Do you know what they are for?
Home Planning	What do you see as the biggest barriers to figure out before going home? What ideas do you have?

Contextual Observation

Another way to identify a need that you could address in speech-language therapy is to actually observe real life activities within your assessment. The idea of contextual observation—or watching someone perform activities within the context they will need to perform them—can be efficient and insightful for understanding why an activity may not be going well, and what intervention may be appropriate to try in therapy.

Why is contextual observation so important? If someone says they are having a hard time making phone calls, we need to know more about that. By observing that activity, we can see what the problem might be. Dialing the number? Finding the phone number? Sequencing the apps to get to the correct spot? Understanding others on the phone call? Not knowing how to repair when others don't understand them? The fastest way to glean all of this information is to actually observe a functional need—something the person needs to do or wants to do. I've found that at the moment someone expresses that something has been difficult—such as making a phone call, finding a baseball game on TV, paying a bill—is a wonderful time to ask them to show me how they are doing that activity. By observing an activity, I have a deeper understanding of why the person is having difficulty in a certain area, and how speech-language therapy can be used to meet that need. This information can also be used as a baseline for functional goal setting. Here is an example of a goal that targets using the television remote: "The client will be able to use the TV remote to navigate to three favorite TV stations with external supports collaboratively created with SLP, compared to baseline of zero TV stations at time of evaluation."

Accessible Communication Materials

As experts in communication, it is vital that we begin to connect those with cognitive-communication disorders with materials that allow them to communicate what is important to them. We may need to use resources and materials that have been developed to support communication with pictures in order to identify values, priorities, and needs. See Table 3–4 for a summary of communication resources that may support communication for discovering functional needs.

Standardized Tests that Point to an Activity

In addition to understanding needs and activities through the nonstandardized portion of assessment, the standardized assessment may also provide you with some valuable information.

Table 3–4. Aphasia-Friendly Resources to Assist with Discovering Functional Needs

Resource	About	Learn More:
Aphasia Access Resource Exchange	Aphasia-friendly resources are shared so you don't have to reinvent the wheel (membership required).	https://www.aphasiaaccess.org/resource-exchange
Aphasia Friendly Resources	This contains 1-page resources for supporting expression in hospital with topics like PEG and CT Scan. There are many free items, some for purchase.	http://www.Aphasiafriendly.co
Aphasia Institute ParticiPics	This includes pictographs and customizable templates designed for people with aphasia, for conversation, participation needs, and education. Free.	https://www.participics.ca/
Australian Aphasia Rehab Pathway	This site contains research guidelines to make your information aphasia-friendly. Free.	http://www.aphasiapathway.com.au/?name=Support-materials-for-people-with-aphasia
Eastern Health Cue Cards in the Community	It includes picture/word support in dozens of languages. They are customizable for category and number of photos on page. Free after entering email address.	https://www.easternhealth.org.au/services/language-services/cue-cards/cue-cards-in-community-languages
Life Interests and Values (LIV) Cards	The site contains research-based black-and-white drawings for people with aphasia to facilitate goal setting, conversations, and more. For purchase.	https://www.med.unc.edu/ahs/sphs/card/resources/liv-cards/ Haley, K., Womack, J., Helm-Estabrooks, N., Caignon, D., & McCulloch, K. (2010)
National Aphasia Association	A personalized Aphasia ID—Free.	http://aphasiaid.com/

Table 3–4. *continued*

Resource	About	Learn More:
UK Stroke Association	This is a workbook-style guide to making information accessible for people with aphasia—Free.	https://www.stroke .org.uk/sites/default/ files/accessible_ information_ guidelines.pdf1_.pdf
UNC Center for Aphasia and Related Disorders: Aphasia-Friendly Print Materials	This contains a bank of student-created aphasia-friendly materials of various topics. You are able to request projects you would like to be made aphasia-friendly by graduate students.	https://www.med.unc .edu/ahs/sphs/card/ resources/aphasia-friendly-printed-material/
Widgit Health Communication Boards	This site includes contains downloadable communication boards with topics like tracheostomy, bedside messages, and more. Many are free, some for cost.	https://widgit-health .com/downloads/for-professionals.htm

As our field moves towards a person-centered approach, re-searchers have recognized that impairment testing alone does not give the full clinical picture. There are some standardized tests available that start to point to activity/participation, either through tasks that are integrative in the skills that they use, or tasks that can be done in a real-life context. For examples of standardized tests that include activity information, see Table 3–5.

Writing Measurable Goals to Meet Functional Needs

As functional needs are discovered in the assessment, it's important to write goals that directly relate to the priority needs. It has been recommended to write SMARTER Goals: Goals that are Shared, Monitored, Accessible, Relevant, Transparent, Evolving, and Relationship-Centered (Hersh, 2012; Hersh, Worrall, Howe,

Table 3–5. Examples of Standardized Tests that Include an Activity Component

Test Name	Author(s)	Details
Arizona Battery for Communication Disorders of Dementia (ABCD)	Bayles, K., & Tomoeda, C., 2005	Used for dementia population, age 15+ Used for differential diagnosis, treatment goals, monitoring progress, planning discharge
Assessment of Language-Related Functional Activities (ALFA)	Baines, K., Martin, A., & McMartin Heeringa, H., 2017	Used for neurologic disorder population, age 16+ Addresses language and cognition
ASHA Quality of Communication Life Scale (ASHA-QCL)	Paul, D., Frattali, C., Holland, A., Thompson, C., Caperton, C., & Slater, S., 2004	Used for adults with communication disorders to measure quality of life. Recommended as a supplement with ASHA-FACS
ASHA Functional Assessment of Communication Skills (ASHA-FACS)	Frattali, C., Thompson, C., Holland, A., Wohl, C., Wenck, C., Slater, S., & Paul, D., 2017	Used with aphasia, TBI, dementia, right brain stroke; Rather than measure impairment, measures how an ADL is affected
Assessment for Living With Aphasia (ALA)	The Aphasia Institute, 2013	Self-report measure; gains perspective of those living with aphasia; Corresponds with WHO-ICF and A-FROM. Includes pictographs for conversation
Behavioral Assessment of Dysexecutive Syndrome (BADS)	Wilson, B., Alderman, N., Burgess, P., Emslie, H., & Evans, J., 1996	Used with brain injury population, age 16 to 87. Predicts everyday problems associated with dysexecutive syndrome.
Communication Abilities of Daily Living (CADL-3)	Holland, A., Fromm, D., & Wozniak, L., 2018	Used with neurogenic communication disorders including stroke, PPA, dementia, TBI, age 18 to 95+.

Table 3–5. *continued*

Test Name	Author(s)	Details
Functional Assessment of Verbal Reasoning and Executive Strategies (FAVRES)	MacDonald, S., 1998	Used with acquired brain injury population, age 18 to 79. Detects subtle cognitive-communication deficits with challenging functional tasks. Scores for accuracy, rationale/reasoning, speed.
Functional Linguistic Communication Inventory (FLCI)	Bayles, K., & Tomoeda, C., 1994	Used with dementia population.
Functional Standardized Touchscreen Assessment of Cognition (FSTAC)	Cognitive Innovations, 2016	At time of writing, this is a screening. It is included because it offers a way to observe functional performance like paying a bill over the phone, grocery shopping, and so forth.
Scales of Cognitive and Communicative Ability in Neurorehabilitation (SCCAN)	Milman, L., & Holland, A., 2012	Used in multiple settings for stroke, Alzheimers, TBI, with language and non-language based disorders; Measures impairment and functional ability with ADLs. Identifies impairment, severity and drafts patient-specific treatment plan.
Student–Functional Assessment of Verbal Reasoning and Executive Strategies (S-FAVRES)	MacDonald, S., 2015	Used with acquired brain injury population, age 12 to 19. Detects subtle cognitive-communication deficits with challenging functional tasks. Scores for accuracy, rationale/reasoning, speed.
Texas Functional Living Scales (TFLS)	Cullum, M., Saine, K., & Weiner, M., 2009	Used for cognitive decline for dementia, age 16 to 90. Focuses on functional skills for time, money, memory, communication, and intended for use in assisted living and nursing homes.

Sherratt, & Davidson, 2012; Worrall, 2019). In what follows, some practical tools that may assist with writing SMARTER goals are discussed.

Goal Attainment Scaling

Goal Attainment Scaling (GAS) is a goal-setting process that is completed with the client and SLP together. Goals and success are defined on a 5-point scale. This allows personalization of many types of goals and progress, and allows "messy" life variables to be characterized within a point system (O'Brien, Schellinger, & Kennedy, 2013; Grant, Ponsford, & Bennett, 2012; Schlosser, 2004). Both qualitative and quantitative factors can be described on the GAS template. Using this process not only helps define a goal from the client's perspective, but also defines success from their point of view. See Figure 3–2 for an example of Goal Attainment Scaling.

Goal Mapping

Goal Mapping is a goal-setting process using a "roadmap." The process starts with the end goal and works backwards so there is a concrete connection between current therapy activities and the final goal (Sohlberg & Turkstra, 2011; Turkstra, 2013). Goal Mapping promotes person-centered care by using a client's end goal as a filter for choosing which therapy activities to address in a hierarchy. Creating the goal map promotes a partnership mentality, and is a concrete reminder to help patients and families clearly see how therapy activities relate to a long-term goal. Creating this goal map can initially be a goal of therapy. Here is an example: "The patient and SLP will complete goal mapping template to assist in education and therapy expectations." As therapy progresses, the goal map can be used for further therapy goals: "As described in goal mapping, the patient will be able to send 2 to 3 word text messages using templates, as part of a larger goal to return to social activities with friends." See Figure 3–3 for an example of Goal Mapping.

Situation: Use of Call Light/Remote (Problem Solving)

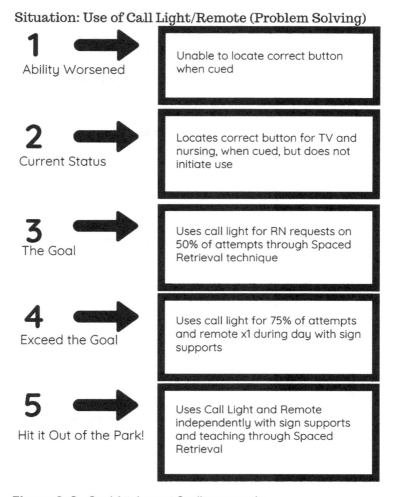

1 ➡ Ability Worsened — Unable to locate correct button when cued

2 ➡ Current Status — Locates correct button for TV and nursing, when cued, but does not initiate use

3 ➡ The Goal — Uses call light for RN requests on 50% of attempts through Spaced Retrieval technique

4 ➡ Exceed the Goal — Uses call light for 75% of attempts and remote x1 during day with sign supports

5 ➡ Hit it Out of the Park! — Uses Call Light and Remote independently with sign supports and teaching through Spaced Retrieval

Figure 3–2. Goal Attainment Scaling example.

Broaden What You Measure

Just as our framework for treatment has broadened beyond simply measuring the impairment, the ways we view real-life functioning offer us many angles to measure participation, success, or improvement.

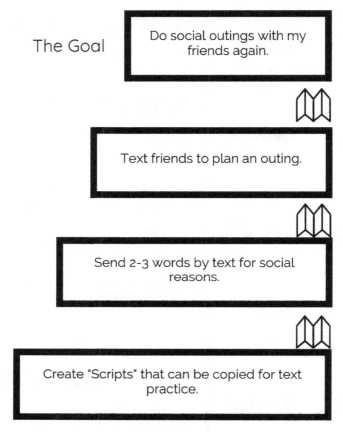

Figure 3–3. Goal Mapping example.

- Skill
- Strategy
- Efficiency
- Education/Knowledge
- Family Support
- Environmental Modification

When identifying a functional need, it can be helpful to determine which one of the areas to measure. It's best to select the area that will make the largest difference in function for the client. Every area of a need does not need to be measured—for example, you may start by tracking strategy use, and then advance to tracking efficiency as time goes on. To see examples of Goal Samples using the methods described above for different medical settings, see Table 3–6.

Case Application

History

Nancy is a 68-year-old woman who has moderate-severe aphasia and is newly wheelchair-bound as a result of a hemorrhagic stroke. She was discharged to assisted living after 2 months of acute care and inpatient rehab. Prior to the stroke, she was healthy and active, living independently, volunteering regularly, and enjoyed hobbies such as choir and traveling. She has a significant other of 30+ years. Nancy was evaluated at her assisted living facility after being discharged from inpatient rehab.

Nonstandardized Assessment

At the start of the assessment, Nancy's significant other did not make any attempts to communicate directly with Nancy and appeared uncomfortable, wanting to leave the room. When he left, Nancy became tearful when asked about communicating with him. I used motivational interviewing techniques: "I can see that you feel frustrated. You're working really hard but he didn't know how to communicate with you. Would that be important for us to spend time on in speech-language therapy? The conversation was continued by my using aphasia-friendly techniques and resources including: ParticiPics (ParticiPics, n.d.), Written words, Supported Conversation for Adults with Aphasia (SCA™) techniques (Supported Conversation for Adults with Aphasia, n.d.), and a setting-specific checklist. We used these techniques to discuss needs in Nancy's new residence, the assisted living unit. Nancy spent a lot of time indicating frustration with not being able to communicate about time, and also food choices.

Table 3–6. "Broaden What You Measure" Goal Samples

Skill	Acute: The patient will use 2+ sentences to explain safe bed transfer.
	Inpatient Rehab: The patient will report name and date of birth for medical questions, using spaced retrieval intervention, after 20-minute delay.
	Home Health: The patient will use follow +4/4 steps to run dishwasher, using systematic instruction and chaining.
	Outpatient: The patient will send an e-mail summary of simulated work meetings with 2 spelling errors or less.
Strategy	Acute: The patient will refer to written phone numbers to make a personal phone call.
	Inpatient Rehab: The patient will independently use self-advocacy script (Can you repeat that?) in a 30-minute session.
	Home Health: The patient will generate 2 strategies to try for home problem-solving scenarios (insurance, banking, pet).
	Outpatient: The patient will create daily to-do list as a strategy for attention and prioritization, 3 times in the coming week.
Efficiency	Acute: The patient will report 2 safety recommendations in hospital in 2 minutes or less.
	Inpatient Rehab: The patient will order meal with picture cues in 5 minutes or less, 50% of the time (baseline 0%).
	Home Health: The patient will generate 6 grandkid names using labels with photos, compared to baseline of 2 names.
	Outpatient: The patient will be able to generate a grocery list using personalized choice aid in 30 minutes or less per tracking log.
Family Support	Acute: The family will demonstrate Supportive Communication techniques x2 during 5-minute conversation.
	Inpatient Rehab: The family will track repetitive questioning behaviors and triggers on log over 4 days, to increase family awareness and support behaviors.
	Home Health: The family will complete recipe modification with 4 recipes after technique is taught by SLP, in order for patient to return to cooking lunches.
	Outpatient: The family will demonstrate "Don't Ask, Just Tell" supportive memory techniques during 5-minute conversation.

Table 3–6. *continued*

Education/ Knowledge	Acute: The patient will verbalize 2 discharge recommendations from the therapy team.
	Inpatient Rehab: The patient will implement knowledge to "minimize distractions" 1 time during 30-minute session.
	Home Health: The patient will implement association memory strategy to recall 3 medication names.
	Outpatient: The patient will select 1 home need to apply goal-plan-do-review framework for home program.
Environmental Modification	Acute: The patient will indicate pain location with enlarged picture and numeric scale.
	Inpatient Rehab: The patient will independently brush teeth using 3-step picture and word sequence on bathroom mirror.
	Home Health: The patient will demonstrate ability to log-in to email using label reminders on computer, with 2 self-corrections or less.
	Outpatient: The patient will improve blood sugar tracking with items set in central location and high-contrast tracking log implemented.

I asked Nancy to show me on a clock, and on her planner, what time we had speech-language therapy today. We figured out that she could accurately recognize numbers and point on a clock or planner, but she was unable to verbalize or write any time or numbers. I asked Nancy to show me what grocery item she needed, and she wheeled over to her bathroom to point to the toilet paper. We didn't make it any further on the needs checklist because the topics we covered were expressed as the highest priority for Nancy. At this point, we attempted a Person-Centered Outcome, and Nancy scored herself on the lowest rating for every item of the Communicative Confidence Rating Scale for Aphasia (CCRSA) (Babbit, Heinemann, Semik, & Cherney, 2011).

Standardized Assessment

We completed the Western Aphasia Battery-Revised (WAB-R™) Bedside Screen (Kertesz, 2006). Nancy scored 64.8/100.

Goal-Setting

Together, we reviewed the needs from the nonstandardized assessment, along with impairments from the standardized assessment. Nancy and I collaboratively agreed to the following goals as needs and priorities for her situation:

- Nancy and her significant other will complete 3 coaching sessions with SLP to learn Supportive Communication for Aphasia (SCA™) techniques.
- Nancy and her significant other will be able to relay and validate 3 pieces of information in 5 minutes (baseline 0 successful transactions).
- Nancy will order breakfast successfully on +5/7 days per week with personalized language aid, tracked by Nancy's report.
- Nancy and SLP will develop a personalized grocery list that can be circled to communicate what items she needs.
- Nancy and SLP will explore planner modification (size, layout, stickers) to improve her ability to indicate time and regain a sense of control with her schedule, and implement 1 modification in 2 weeks.
- Nancy will demonstrate improved communication confidence in daily activities, as measured by improved rating on the CCRSA (baseline score 0/100).

Conclusion

The Life Participation approach is a mindset for therapy that broadens the way we can address real-life needs in speech-language therapy from the very first visit. This person-centered approach can improve outcomes, patient satisfaction, efficiency with meeting goals, and is consistent with our best practices in adult medical speech-language therapy. In order to discover functional needs, we have tools such as motivational interviewing, person-centered outcomes, needs checklists, and contextual observation. With these tools, we become able to set holistic goals for therapy that impact more than skills, strategies, or efficiency: Both our therapy and time can have a positive impact on individuals' ability to participate in society, as well as their own confidence and well-being.

References

American Speech-Language-Hearing Association (n.d.). *Practice portal.* Retrieved from http://www.asha.org/Practice-Portal/Clinical-Topics/ *Assessment of Living with Aphasia.* (2013). The Aphasia Institute.

Babbitt, E. M., & Cherney, L. R. (2010). Communication confidence in persons with aphasia. *Topics in Stroke Rehabilitation, 17*(3), 214–223.

Babbitt, E., Heinemann, A., Semik, P., & Cherney, L. (2011). Psychometric properties of the Communication Confidence Rating Scale for Aphasia (CCRSA): Phase 2. *Aphasiology, 25,* 727–735.

Baines, K., Martin, A., & McMartin Heeringa, H. (2017). *Assessment of Language-Related Functional Activities.* Pro-Ed.

Bayles, K., & Tomoeda, C. (1994). *Functional Linguistic Communication Inventory.* Austin, TX: Pro-Ed.

Bayles, K., & Tomoeda, C. (2005). *Arizona Battery for Communication Disorders of Dementia.* Austin, TX: Pro-Ed.

Coelho, C., Ylvisaker, M., & Turkstra, L. (2005). Nonstandardized assessment approaches for individuals with traumatic brain injury. *Seminars in Speech and Language, 26*(4), 223–241.

Cullum, M., Saine, K., & Weiner, M. (2009). *Texas Functional Living Scale.* Pearson Assessments.

Davenport, S., Dickinson, A., & Minns Lowe, C. (2019). Therapy-based exercise from the perspective of adult patients: A qualitative systematic review conducted using an ethnographic approach. *Clinical Rehabilitation, 33*(12), 1963–1977.

Dilollo, A., & Favreau, C. (2010). Person-centered care in speech and language therapy. *Seminars in Speech and Language, 31*(2), 90–97.

Dutzi, I, Schwenk, M., Kirchner, M, Bauer, J., & Hauer, K. (2019). "What would you like to achieve?" Goal-setting in patients with dementia in geriatric rehabilitation. *BMC Geriatrics, 19,* 280.

Epstein, R., Fiscella, K., Lesser, C., & Strange, K. (2010). Why the nation needs a policy push on patient-centered healthcare. *Health Affairs, 29*(8), 1489–1495.

Frattali, C., Thompson, C., Holland, A., Wohl, C., Wenck, C., Slater, S., & Paul, D. (2017). *ASHA Functional Assessment of Communication Skills.* Rockville, MD: American Speech-Language-Hearing Association.

Functional Standardized Touchscreen Assessment of Cognition (FSTAC) (2016). Cognitive Innovations.

Grant, M., Ponsford, J., & Bennett, P. (2012). The application of goal management training to aspects of financial management in individuals with traumatic brain injury. *Neuropsychological Rehabilitation, 22*(6), 852–873.

Haley, K., Womack, J., Helm-Estabrooks, N., Caignon, D., & McCulloch, K. (2010). *The life interests and values cards.* Chapel Hill, NC: University of North Carolina Department of Allied Health Sciences.

Hersh, D., Worrall, L., Howe, T., Sherratt, S., & Davidson, B. (2012). SMARTER goal setting in aphasia rehabilitation. *Aphasiology, 26*(2), 220–233.

Holland, A. L., Fromm, D., & Wozniak, L. (2018). *CADL-3: Communication Abilities of Daily Living* (3rd ed.). Austin, TX: Pro-Ed.

Kagan, A. L., Simmons-Mackie, N., Rowland, A., Huijbregts, M., Shumway, E., McEwen, S., . . . Sharp, S. (2008). Counting what counts: A framework for capturing real-life outcomes of aphasia intervention. *Aphasiology, 22*(3), 258–280.

Kagan, A., & Simmons-Mackie, N. (2007). Beginning with the end: Outcome-driven assessment and intervention with life participation in mind. *Topics in Language Disorders, 27*(4), 309–317.

Kertesz, A. (2006). *Western Aphasia Battery (WAB™)—Revised (WAB-R™).* San Antonio, TX: Pearson Education.

LeBlanc J., Hayden M., & Paulman R. (2000). A comparison of neuropsychological and situational assessment for predicting employability after closed head injury. *Journal of Head Trauma Rehabilitation, 15*, 1022–1040.

LPAA Project Group: Chapey, R., Duchan, J. F., Elman, R. J., Garcia, L. J., Kagan, A., Lyon, J., & Simmons-Mackie, N. (2000). Life participation approach to aphasia: A statement of values for the future. *ASHA Leader, 5*(3), 4–6. https://doi.org/10.1044/leader.FTR.05032000.4

MacDonald, S. (2015). *Student—Functional Assessment of Verbal Reasoning and Executive Strategies.* Ontario, Canada: CCD Publishing.

MacDonald, S. (1998). *Functional Assessment of Verbal Reasoning and Executive Strategies.* Ontario, Canada: CCD Publishing.

MacFarlane, L. (2012). Motivational interviewing: Practical strategies for speech-language pathologists and audiologists. *Canadian Journal of Speech-Language Pathology and Audiology, 36*(1), 8–16.

Milman, L., & Holland, A. (2012). *Scales of Cognitive and Communicative Ability in Neurorehabilitation.* Austin, TX: Pro-Ed.

O'Brien, K., Schellinger, S., & Kennedy, M. (2013, November). *Tracking self-regulation goals using goal-attainment scaling for individuals with traumatic brain injuries* [PowerPoint slides]. Presented to the American Speech-Language-Hearing Association Convention,

Chicago, IL. Retrieved from http://www.asha.org/events/convention/handouts/2013/5080-obrien/

ParticiPics (n.d.). Developed by the Aphasia Institute, Toronto, Canada. Retrieved from https://www.participics.ca/

Paul, D., Frattali, C., Holland, A., Thompson, C., Caperton, C., & Slater, S. (2004). *ASHA Quality of Communication Life Scale.* Rockville, MD: American Speech-Language-Hearing Association.

Schlosser, R. (2004). Goal attainment scaling as a clinical measurement technique in communication disorders: A critical review. *Journal of Communication Disorders, 37,* 217–239.

Sohlberg, M., & Turkstra, L. (2011). *Optimizing cognitive rehabilitation.* New York, NY: Guilford Press.

Supported Conversation for Adults with Aphasia (SCA™). (n.d.). Developed by the Aphasia Institute, Toronto, Canada. Retrieved from https://www.aphasia.ca/communicative-access-sca/

Torrence, J. M., Baylor, C. R., Yorkston, K. M., & Spencer, K. A. (2016). Addressing communicative participation in treatment planning for adults: A survey of U.S. speech-language pathologists. *American Journal of Speech-Language Pathology, 25*(3), 355–370.

Turkstra, Lyn. (2013). Inpatient cognitive rehab: Is it time for a change? *Journal of Head Trauma Rehabilitation, 28*(4), 332–336.

Wilson, B., Alderman, N., Burgess, P., Emslie, H., & Evans, J. (1996). *Behavioral Assessment of Dysexecutive Syndrome.* Upper Saddle River, NJ: Pearson.

World Health Organization (WHO). (2001). *International classification of functioning, disability, and health (ICF).* Geneva, Switzerland: Author.

Whyte, J., & Barrett, A. M. (2013). Advancing the evidence base of rehabilitation treatments: A developmental approach. *Physical Medicine & Rehabilitation, 93*(80), S101–110.

Worrall, L., Sherratt, S., Rogers, P., Howe, T., Hersh, D., Ferguson, A., & Davidson, B. (2011). What people with aphasia want: Their goals according to the ICF. *Aphasiology, 25*(3), 309–322.

Worrall, L. (2019). The seven habits of highly effective aphasia therapists: The perspective of people living with aphasia. *International Journal of Speech–Language Pathology, 21*(5), 438–447.

Wray, F., Clarke, D., & Forster, A. (2019). How do stroke survivors with communication difficulties manage life after stroke in the first year? A qualitative study. *International Journal of Language & Communication Disorders, 54*(5), 814–827.

Yorkston, K., Baylor, C., & Britton, D. (2017). Speech vs speaking: The experiences of people with Parkinson's Disease and implications for intervention. *American Journal of Speech-Language Pathology, 26,* 561–568.

THE ROLE OF THE ENVIRONMENT

SUPPORTING LANGUAGE, COMMUNICATION, AND PARTICIPATION

Thomas W. Sather and Tami J. Howe

Communication is, by definition, interactive; therefore the environment is crucial to improvement in function for individuals with communication disorders."

—Threats, 2000, p. xvii

Introduction

As described so astutely in the opening chapter, the consequences of aphasia require the social imperative—a comprehensive approach to aphasia rehabilitation. One key component of this approach involves directly addressing the environment in order to enhance language, communication, participation, and overall quality of life. This focus on the environment aligns directly with one of the core values of the Life Participation Approach to Aphasia (LPAA; LPAA Project Group, 2000, p. 3): "environmental factors (EFs) are intervention targets." Environmental factors include everything and everyone external to the person with aphasia (PWA). Positive EFs, or facilitators, such as the availability of trained conversation partners, accessible written information, or communicatively supportive conversation groups, enable the PWA to participate more fully in their everyday life. Conversely, negative EFs, or barriers (e.g., a spouse who does not allow the PWA sufficient time to formulate a response), hinder participation.

Environmental factors are important to address in order to enhance health and well-being in clients with a variety of health conditions (Woolf & Aron, 2013) including aphasia (O'Halloran, Carragher, & Foster, 2017). Furthermore, EFs can play a key role in living successfully with aphasia (Manning, MacFarlane, Hickey, & Franklin, 2019).

In this chapter, we emphasize the feasibility and importance of environmental assessment and interventions, regardless of treatment setting, payor source, extent of aphasia, or degree of chronicity. It does not require a "novel" environment. Sometimes we hear from others that "an environmental approach may work in a university, but not in a clinic/hospital/nursing home setting" or that "this only works at an aphasia camp . . . we can't do that here because of X." Just because you work in, for example, a brick-and-mortar medical institution does not mean you cannot address the environment. Incorporating the environment involves identifying the everyday environments in which the PWA needs to communicate, which may include community interactions with staff and patrons at restaurants, church, synagogue, or coffee shops. It may also include interacting with health care staff or cafeteria workers at a hospital or skilled nursing facility in which the person is residing, either temporarily or permanently.

Specifically, we suggest that aphasia service providers (e.g., clinicians, aphasia program directors, aphasiologists, researchers, medical staff, etc.) consider the following "Five E's of the

Environment" as part of the Social Imperative for aphasia rehabilitation:

1. **Environments** are driven by the PWA and family members
2. **Enhance** facilitators and reduce barriers
3. **Enrich** the communicative environment
4. **Embed** challenge intentionally
5. **Evaluate** the environmental intervention.

Environments Are Driven by the Person with Aphasia and Family Members

We argue that a fundamental principle of the social imperative is that the PWA and their family need to drive the environment. Although it may be easy to depend on our own perceptions and experiences as speech-language pathologists (SLPs) to set rehabilitation goals for our clients, such reliance ignores the expertise and priorities of those with aphasia and their family members. As a result, SLP goals may not align with those of the PWA (Rohde, Townley-O'Neill, Trendall, Worrall, & Cornwall, 2012). Therefore, we advocate that the SLP work collaboratively with the client and their family to identify and target the settings and EFs which are the most important to them. One way to do this is to follow the principles of SMARTER goal-setting (Hersh, Worrall, Howe, Sherratt, & Davidson, 2012) to ensure that there is shared-decision making. This approach can be implemented by conducting a semi-structured interview with conversational supports (Hersh et al., 2012) or using a tool such as the Assessment for Living with Aphasia (ALA; Kagan et al., 2011) or the FOURC model (Haley, Cunningham, Barry, & de Riesthal, 2019).

Enhance Facilitators and Reduce Barriers

Once the most relevant settings and life areas have been identified, the SLP can collaborate with the PWA and family to target the key EFs within these contexts. Positive EFs, or facilitators, support the PWA's participation (e.g., aphasia-friendly appointment cards) and need to be enhanced or introduced, whereas negative EFs, or barriers, hinder participation (e.g., clinic receptionist who speaks too quickly to a PWA) and need to be reduced or removed. EFs can be grouped into three broad categories:

a. Other people EFs (which corresponds to the "Support and relationships" and "Attitudes" chapters of the International Classification of Functioning, Disability, and Health (ICF) (World Health Organization, 2001))
b. Physical EFs (which corresponds to the "Products and technology" and "Natural environment and human-made changes to environment" ICF chapters)
c. Service, system, and policy EFs (which corresponds to the "Services, systems, and policies" ICF chapter).

Some of the tools listed in the "Evaluate the environmental intervention" section later in this chapter can help clinicians identify the key EFs to focus on within each of these categories.

Other People Environmental Factors

Because communication typically involves at least two individuals, *other people EFs* are often the most important factors on which the SLP can focus. These *other people EFs* include other people's knowledge about aphasia (e.g., disability shuttle bus driver knowing what aphasia is), their skills for communicating with the PWA (e.g., friend printing key words while speaking to support a conversation), and their attitudes towards the PWA (e.g., shop assistant respecting and treating the PWA as a competent adult). EFs in this category are often targeted through communication partner training (CPT), in which people around the PWA learn strategies to support the individual's communication participation. As highlighted in Chapter One, the idea of training the partners without aphasia to support the communication of a PWA is a "cornerstone" of the Social Imperative for aphasia rehabilitation.

Partner training programs can be categorized into generic and dyad-focused approaches (Saldert, Jensen, Blom Johansson, & Simmons-Mackie, 2018). Generic CPT involves training partners to communicate with a variety of people with different types of aphasia, usually in a specific setting (e.g., physical therapists, radiology technicians, food service and other health care workers, bus drivers, stroke organization volunteers, home care assistants). One well-known generic approach, Supported Conversation for Adults with Aphasia (SCA™; Kagan, 1998), trains communication partners to use strategies to acknowledge (e.g., using a natural adult tone of voice) and reveal the competence of a PWA (e.g., encouraging the PWA to gesture, point, write part of the word, or draw if they have difficulties expressing an idea) [See "An Introduction to supported Conversation for Adults with Aphasia (SCA™) Self-Directed Learning Module at http://www.aphasia.ca for online resources]. Other examples of generic approaches include a program for improving the communication of health care professionals in inpatient stroke rehabilitation units (Horton, Lane, & Shiggins, 2016) and a program for improving medical students' interactions with individuals with a variety of communication disorders including aphasia (Burns, Baylor, Morris, McNalley, & Yorkston, 2012).

To be most effective, generic CPT should be supplemented with individualized information about the unique communication needs of specific individuals with aphasia who will be interacting with the partner. For example, after providing generic CPT in a long-term care facility, the clinician could work with a nursing assistant to develop a personalized communication care plan for a person with a more severe aphasia (Page & Rowles, 2016).

In contrast to generic approaches, dyad-focused CPT (Saldert et al., 2018) targets behaviors which are specific to a familiar communication partner (e.g., family member, friend, rehabilitation assistant, or volunteer) and a PWA. This training includes individualizing components of a generic approach such as SCA™ to a specific PWA and their partner (Cunningham & Ward, 2003), as well as using a specific approach such as Better Conversations with Aphasia (BCA; Beeke et al., 2013). BCA uses video recordings of natural conversations between the communication partner and the PWA to train specific communication behaviors (e.g., wife asking the PWA fewer "test" questions, for which she already knows the answer; husband with aphasia writing or gesturing when he cannot say a word). The feedback provided by the video recordings helps the dyad to gain more insight into their communication behaviors. This program provides extensive free online resources including video recorded examples of effective and less effective communication interactions and handouts for family members and people with aphasia (https://www.ucl.ac.uk/short-courses/search-courses/better-conversations-aphasia-e-learning-resource). Instead of using video feedback, two other dyad-focused approaches, Conversational coaching (Holland, 2008; Hopper, Holland, & Rwega, 2002) and Aphasia Couples' Therapy (Boles, 2009), involve the SLP coaching a familiar partner and the PWA to use their individualized communication strategies during real-time conversations.

Communication partner training can seem deceptively simple and straightforward (Holland, 2008). However, giving a handout with a list of strategies to a family member or health care worker is insufficient. In both generic and dyad-focused CPT, it is important that the SLP demonstrate the strategies and provide the partners with ample opportunities to practice the skills with feedback (McGilton et al., 2011). Preferably, this training should include an experiential learning component with face-to-face practice with an individual with aphasia (McGilton et al., 2011) and, where possible, take place in more naturalistic settings (Simmons-Mackie, Raymer, & Cherney, 2016).

Physical Environmental Factors

Physical EFs include tangible resources used to support conversations, reading, and writing (Simmons-Mackie, King, & Beukelman, 2013), as well as other auditory, visual, and spatial factors. Examples of a range of physical facilitators which a SLP might consider focusing on are provided in Table 4–1. (Note: for an extensive list of additional physical facilitators see Simmons-Mackie et al., 2013).

After appropriate physical facilitators for supporting conversations, reading, or writing have been identified, clinicians can provide those with aphasia and their key communication partners with numerous guided opportunities to practice using the resources in naturalistic situations. Failure to do this may result in

Table 4–1. Physical Facilitators

Examples of Physical Facilitators for Supporting Conversations

- Paper, pencils, and felt-tip markers
- "Yes, no, and other" cards
- Simplified rating scales (e.g., for the PWA to respond regarding preferences and opinions such as satisfaction with a particular TV show or football coach; Garrett & Lasker, 2013)
- Presence of the object being communicated about (e.g., PWA taking an example of the type of nail he needs to the hardware store to show the shop assistant; Howe, Worrall, & Hickson, 2008a)
- Photographs, calendars, maps, low technology and other resources (e.g., ParticiPics—the free, searchable pictographic database from the Aphasia Institute: https://www.participics.ca/)
- Aphasia identification wallet card for educating unfamiliar communication partners
- Specific message cards (e.g., key details about lottery ticket numbers, directions for a taxi driver, how the PWA likes their coffee; Garrett & Lasker, 2013)
- Personalized communication books and low-tech visual scene displays (Hux, Buechter, Wallace, & Weissling, 2010)
- Remnant books (e.g., collection of meaningful objects from PWA's daily life such as a college football game ticket stub, restaurant business card, movie receipt, art exhibit brochure; Ho, Weiss, Garrett, & Lloyd, 2005)
- Smartphone and tablet apps (e.g., PWA or communication partner using photos, video clips, calendar, map, notes, and other native apps to support conversations)
- High-technology augmentative and alternative communication (AAC) devices [e.g., speech-generating device with a preprogrammed message for answering the telephone: "Hello, this is Jenny. Please ask me questions that can be answered with a yes or no. Please speak clearly and slowly." (Garrett & Lasker, 2013); visual scene displays on a high-tech device (Beukelman, Hux, Dietz, McKelvery, & Weissling, 2015)].

Examples of Physical Facilitators for Supporting Reading

- Aphasia-friendly written materials (e.g., hospital menus, physical therapy homework handouts; see Rose, Worrall, Hickson, & Hoffmann, 2011 for a list of aphasia-friendly content and design variables to consider).
- Aphasia-friendly or simplified language websites (e.g., Simple English Wikipedia; News websites with simplified language websites such as: https://newsela.com/rules/latest; http://talkpathnews.aphasia.com/ https://www.newsinlevels.com/)
- Aphasia-friendly book resources (e.g., Book Connection™ Aphasia Book Club at the Aphasia Center of California; www.aphasiacenter.net/ programs/aphasia-book-club/)

continues

Table 4–1. *continued*

- Audiobooks
- Large-print books
- Text to speech conversion system on electronic devices (Knollman-Porter et al., 2019)
- Vocabulary simplification apps (e.g., Rewordify.com)
- Aphasia-friendly brochures and documents for tourist attractions and outdoor environmental activities (Bernstein-Ellis & Avent, 2013)
- Aphasia-friendly signage (e.g. color-coded; inclusion of clear photos or icons; Howe et al., 2008a)

Examples of Physical Facilitators for Supporting Written Expression

- Aphasia-friendly forms (e.g., aphasia-friendly registration form for an exercise group at a stroke organization; Howe et al., 2008a)
- Personalized writing templates with examples of phrases to choose from (e.g., for copying text messages, e-mails, cards, or letters; Garrett & Lasker, 2013)
- Personalized written resources (e.g., multiple copies of a personalized grocery list in which the PWA can circle the items needed each week; Garrett & Lasker, 2013)
- Speaking to dictation, word prediction, and spelling and grammar checking functions on apps
- Personalized everyday writing apps (e.g., photo-based grocery list apps, barcode scanner apps for making lists)
- Journal template (e.g., structured template to document daily activities, observations, and feelings using photos, clippings, notes, and/or drawings; Simmons-Mackie, 2008; Martin, Thompson, & Worrall, 2007)
- Aphasia Union Netherlands e-mail program (Al Mahmud & Martens, 2016)

Examples of Auditory, Visual, and Spatial Physical Facilitators

- Reduced background noise/Quiet environment
- Clear sound quality on public address systems (e.g., at an airport or public transit station; Howe et al. 2008a)
- Reduced visual distractions (Howe et al. 2008a)
- Merchandise set up in a shop/café so the PWA can point to or independently obtain the item instead of having to request it (e.g., PWA choosing to go to a bakery where muffins are in a glass display case which they can point to; Alary Gauvreau, Kairy, Mazer, Guindon, & Le Dorze, 2018; Howe, Worrall, & Hickson, 2008b)
- Aphasia-friendly resources which are physically available on the hospital ward for communicating about health related information (Kagan & Le Blanc, 2002)
- Seating configuration in a residential facility that is conducive for interaction between residents (Lubinski, 2011)

the PWA and family members not using these resources in everyday life (Garrett & Lasker, 2013). In addition, the clinician should encourage the PWA to be more accountable for their role in using the resources and other strategies to maximize communication effectiveness during conversations. For example, there will be times when the clinician can point out to the PWA that they could be trying to draw, or find a relevant photo on their smartphone, or use another effective strategy to help overcome a communication breakdown.

Service, System, and Policy Environmental Factors

Service, system, and policy EFs involve a variety of intangible factors (e.g., communicatively accessible services, accessibility regulations) which influence the participation of a PWA. Facilitators within this category include small-scale service improvements that clinicians could introduce into their practice, such as working with a PWA and their family to set up a community support team (CST; Silverman, 2011). A CST member might be a friend from a club, church, or workplace who is interested in helping the PWA poststroke, but is unsure what to do. The SLP could train the CST member to become an effective communication partner for the PWA and then help them to support the PWA to participate in an activity that they are interested in (e.g. photography, visiting art galleries, gardening). If appropriate individuals within the PWA's own social network are unavailable, the SLP could provide dyad-focused CPT for a volunteer. The volunteer could then support the PWA to participate in a leisure, social, or volunteer activity of their choice such as taking a floral arranging class or volunteering at the food bank (Lyon et al., 1997). These types of facilitators ensure that the PWA has opportunities for meaningful supported participation because as Simmons-Mackie (2008, p. 304) stated, "Without opportunities to communicate, improved language is a trivial accomplishment."

Many *service, system, and policy EFs* operate at the organizational level. In order to modify them, the SLP may need to collaborate with multiple stakeholders such as managers, other health professionals, and volunteers, in addition to individuals with aphasia and their family members. Although these types of initiatives may be initially time consuming, in the long run, they may result in a sustainable positive impact on the participation of multiple clients with aphasia. Examples of some service, system, and policy facilitators reported in the literature are highlighted in Table 4–2.

Table 4–2. Examples of Service, System, and Policy Facilitators

Examples of Service Facilitators
• Inpatient or outpatient aphasia mentor scheme (Coles & Snow, 2011; Lawrie, Hobson, & Tyson, 2007)
• Communicatively accessible aphasia conversation group led by a skilled facilitator (Elman, 2007; Simmons-Mackie, Elman, Holland, & Damico, 2007)
• A group of people with aphasia can be supported by an SLP to set up their own peer-led aphasia coffee groups (Tregea & Brown, 2013)
• Virtual conversation groups (Walker & Jacques, 2016)
• Accessible aphasia groups which focus on shared interests such as book, music, drama, advocacy, and public speaking (e.g., Aphasia Book Club at the Aphasia Center of California; Cherney, Oehring, Whipple, & Rubenstein, 2011; Plourde et al., 2019; Tarrant et al., 2016)
• Supporting well-being through PEeR Befriending (SUPERB) Scheme (Behn et al., 2019)
• Communicatively accessible book club led by a trained librarian (Henriksson & Laakso, 2019)
• Communicatively accessible art museum project (Duchan, Jennings, Barrett, & Butler, 2006)
• Aphasia-friendly psychological support services (Thomas et al., 2016)
• Aphasia camps (e.g., Kim, Ruelling, Garcia, & Kajner, 2017; Hoepner, Clark, Sather, & Knutson, 2012)
• Aphasia cruises (e.g., "Cruise for a Cause" via Voices of Hope for Aphasia; "Aphasia Cruises" via the Aphasia Recovery Connection)
• Aphasia centers (e.g., Simmons-Mackie & Holland, 2011; Elman, 2016)
• Professional language interpreters/communication intermediaries who are trained to support people with communication difficulties such as aphasia to participate in various community activities (e.g., health appointments, recreational classes; Larsson & Thoren-Jonsson, 2007; Rautakoski, 2014)
• Aphasia advocacy organizations (e.g., Aphasia Access, Aphasia Recovery Connection, Aphasia United, National Aphasia Association)

Table 4–2. *continued*

Examples of System Facilitators
• Implementation of a communicatively accessible capacity evaluation (CACE) process (tool + training) to help health care professionals determine whether or not people with communication disabilities have the capacity to decide where they shall live (Carling-Rowland, Black, McDonald, & Kagan, 2014) • Implementation of an ongoing generic CPT program for health care workers in a large hospital inpatient stroke ward (Jensen et al., 2015) • Implementation of a dyad-focused CPT program for family members across multiple rehabilitation centers (Wielaert, van de Sandt-Koenderman, Dammers, & Sage, 2018) • Implementation of communicative access projects in an acute care, a rehabilitation, and a long-term care setting (Simmons-Mackie et al., 2007; O'Halloran, Lee, Rose, & Liamputtong, 2014) • Development of aphasia-friendly emergency and disaster planning information (Carney, Elman, Rome, & Scheiner, 2019)
Examples of Policy Facilitators
• Communication access standards for identifying communication-friendly businesses (Solarsh & Johnson, 2017) • Accessible Transportation for Persons with Disabilities Regulations (e.g., requiring transportation providers to meet the communication needs of travelers with disabilities; Government of Canada, Canada Transportation Act, 2019)

Enrich the Communicative Environment

Enriching communicative environments is another important principle for SLPs to consider. Rich communicative environments may enhance clients' well-being and support active learning through repeated meaningful engagement in communicative interactions (Duff, Gallegos, Cohen, & Tranel, 2013). Although there is no single optimal environment, characteristics of rich communicative environments include *complexity, voluntariness,* and *quality* (Hengst, Duff, & Jones, 2019).

Rich communicative environments leverage the *complexity* of multiple participants and activities, incorporating varied communicative modalities (e.g., PWA encouraged to use a variety of resources such as speech, gestures, and/or a smartphone to communicate a message) and roles (e.g., switching between being a storyteller and a listener). This complexity provides each person with aphasia multiple ways to achieve their goals and participate within the environment.

The characteristic of *voluntariness* highlights the PWA's right to make choices about how they participate in the environment. For example, in a conversation group, each PWA would voluntarily choose when or whether to contribute to a topic, as typically occurs during authentic conversations, rather than taking turns around the table (Simmons-Mackie et al., 2007).

Finally, the characteristic of *quality* refers to the individual's positive affective experience of a communicative environment. The perception of a quality experiences will vary depending on the person and the moment in time, rather than being a "one size fits all" (Hengst et al., 2019). This characteristic therefore reinforces the importance of ensuring that the PWA and their family drive the environment. It also highlights the need to provide a range of novel as well as familiar activities for people with aphasia to choose from in group settings such as aphasia centers.

Embed Challenge Intentionally

Enriched communicative environments provide challenging and meaningful opportunities for individuals with aphasia. Essential to such environments is the presence of challenge. Without challenge, there is little opportunity for growth, whether with or without aphasia. However, the environmental challenge needs to be scaffolded so that it presents difficulty, but is not so difficult as to overwhelm. This optimal balance of skill and challenge has been called "flow," a term originally coined by positive psychologist Mihaly Csikszentmihalyi (1975). When someone is in flow, " . . . attention is fully invested in the task at hand, and the person functions at his or her fullest capacity" (Csikszent-mihalyi, Abuhamdeh, & Nakamura, 2014, p. 230). The importance of flow, in which challenge slightly exceeds skill, has been implicated in the promotion of physical and social well-being among individuals with disabilities (Delle Fave & Massimini, 2004), and has also been emphasized as an important aspect of a strengths-based approach to counseling and engagement for those with aphasia (Holland & Nelson, 2020). The importance of flow has been studied among a wide range of populations including athletes, artists, and individuals with communication impairments, including aphasia (Lyon et al., 1997; Sather, Howe, Nelson & Lagerwey, 2017).

In order to attain flow experiences, an optimal balance of skill and challenge is required. In contrast, when a task is too challenging (e.g., watching a YouTube cooking video of a chef who talks fast) it leaves a person feeling overwhelmed and more likely to abandon it. A task that is too easy may become boring or mundane (e.g., a person with a very mild reading difficulty as the result of aphasia reading an oversimplified aphasia-friendly paragraph on cooking), and may result in boredom or apathy. Without adequate challenge, flow experiences are unachievable. Too often, we as clinicians may make the error, albeit well-intentioned, of attempting to make an "aphasia-friendly" environment by reducing/eliminating challenges when in reality, we may be erring by removing or reducing *too much* of the challenge. Instead, using the flow framework, there are times when we need to optimize the environment to explicitly embrace and embed challenge at an optimal level that does not overwhelm. Such environments capitalize on the growth that results from such an appropriately challenging, demanding environment. In our 2017 study (Sather et al.), we used a customized, aphasia-friendly iOS app with individuals with aphasia to better understand their levels of day-to-day challenge, as well as flow. Low challenge scenarios were more frequently associated with boredom or apathy as were environments with a perceived reduction in communication complexity (Sather et al., 2017). Such findings parallel the recommendations of Hengst et al. (2019), referenced earlier, that encourage optimizing and enhancing *complexity* as part of an enriched environment.

Evaluate the Environmental Intervention

Clinicians can use a variety of tools to evaluate the overall effectiveness of the environmental intervention. Participation is the ultimate outcome for LPAA, and is closely intertwined with environmental factors. Therefore, SLPs need to evaluate the impact of the intervention on the PWA's participation while also evaluating the EFs. Furthermore, because data collected in contrived settings might not translate to real-life contexts, as much as possible, evaluation should focus on authentic, naturalistic situations. Examples of assessments for identifying EFs and evaluating environmental interventions are presented in Table 4–3.

Case Study

This chapter will conclude with a case example that highlights the Five E's of the Environment:

Environments are driven by those with aphasia and their family members; Enhance facilitators and reduce barriers; Enrich the communicative environment; Embed challenge intentionally; and Evaluate the environmental intervention.

This particular scenario involved the planning and implementation of a regional weekend aphasia event hosted by the local aphasia group. This event was based on the principles of project-based interventions (Behn, Marshall, Togher, & Cruice, 2019) and provided an opportunity to collaboratively create a meaningful, enriched communicative environment.

First, the aphasia group members drove the environment. The idea was posited and developed by the group with only a few budgetary and timing stipulations for hosting the event. Beyond that, it was entirely up to the group. Over the course of group sessions, discussions, and debates, the group arrived on a consensus for the keynote speaker and topic, as well as an additional medical staff person to answer questions the group had generated. The group planned and arranged logistics and food for a fantastic cookout at an area nature preserve in the evening.

Table 4–3. Examples of Environmental and Participation Evaluation Tools

Examples of Assessments—Other People EFs
• Measure of Skill in Supported Conversation and Measure of Level of Participation in Conversation (Kagan et al., 2004)
• Supporting Partners of People with Aphasia in Relationships and Conversation (SPPARC) Assessment (Lock, Wilkinson, & Bryan, 2001)
• Friendship Scale (Hawthorne, 2006). Includes six questions for assessing an individual's perception of social support (e.g., "During the past 4 weeks: I had someone to share my feelings with: Almost always, Most of the time, About half of the time, Occasionally, Not at all.")
• Social Networks: A Communication Inventory for Individuals with Complex Communication Needs and Their Communication Partners (Blackstone & Hunt-Berg, 2003). Includes interviews and observations to obtain information about number and categories of communication partners, communication modalities, topics, and preferences
• Stroke Social Network Scale (Northcott & Hilari, 2013). Assesses the social network of individuals with or without aphasia during the first 6 months poststroke. Includes satisfaction with social network, children, relatives, friends, and groups
• Convoy /Social Network Analysis (Antonucci & Akiyama, 1987, as described for individuals with aphasia in Cruice, Worrall, & Hickson, 2006). Uses three concentric circles for PWA to separate people on the basis of how close they are in relationship to them

Examples of Assessments—Physical EFs
• Multimodal Communication Screening Task for Persons with Aphasia (Garrett & Lasker, 2005)

Examples of Assessments—Multiple EFs and Participation
• Communicative Profiling System (Simmons-Mackie & Damico, 1996). Includes systematic observation of PWA in an authentic naturalistic setting and interviews with key informants
• Assessment for Living with Aphasia (Kagan et al., 2011). Includes a number of questions which specifically focus on EFs, while others focus on participation
• Communicative Access Measure for Stroke (Kagan, Simmons-Mackie, Victor, & Chan, 2017). Evaluates overall communicative access in healthcare settings: (1) institutional level survey; (2) health care staff survey; (3) patient satisfaction survey
• Inpatient Functional Communication Inventory – Environmental Questionnaires (The Overall, The Ward, The Hospital, The External Agencies; O'Halloran, Worrall, Toffolo, & Code, 2020)

Environmental facilitators were enhanced and environmental barriers were reduced in the process of planning and carrying out the project. When searching for lodging options for out-of-town guests, one aphasia group member used speech-to-text strategies to search the World Wide Web (an example of *Physical Facilitators for Supporting Written Expression* listed earlier in Table 4–1). Additionally, the group reviewed and used aphasia-friendly text layout templates to create invitations, logistical information, and a schedule (an example of *Physical Facilitators for Supporting Reading* listed earlier in Table 4–1). The overall model, concept, and paradigm for the hosted event was a *Service Facilitator* (see Table 4–2), providing authentic opportunities for peer-led interactions and collaborations in pursuit of meaningful engagement. During the guest speaker presentation and discussion, as well as during the other small group discussions and interactions, *Physical Facilitators for Supporting Conversations* (see Table 4–1) were always present, including paper and markers, rating scales, and low- and high-tech pictographic resources.

The planning process, and the event itself, incorporated concepts of **enriched communicative environments** to support opportunities for active learning and co-construction of socially complex, collaborative engagement. Enriched communicative environments provide layers of complexity through multiple participants and activities, as well as a multitude of communicative demands. The hosted event described here contained multiple sets and types of participants—ranging from individuals with aphasia and care partners who attended our group, to individuals with aphasia and care partners who were outside of our group network. Information inquiries, scheduling, and confirmation emails were not simulations or role plays. Rather, they were authentic interactions between group members and area businesses, community members, and service providers.

There were multiple occurrences of **intentionally embedded challenge**. Throughout the course of the planning, we intentionally eliminated student involvement for all but a small number of specific tasks. Although there is certainly value in student involvement, we limited it due to growing concerns that group members were deferring to the student clinicians to accomplish some of the tasks that the group members them-selves could accomplish. Indeed, such dependency was evident in a particularly exasperating period of the event planning, when one of the group members exclaimed in exasperation "Where are the students??!!" It became clear that a default mode to challenge was often to solicit others to do it—others without aphasia. In keeping with principles of challenge, providing overwhelming challenge is not effective, and thus, scaffolding was used to support when necessary.

This experience also provided insights and an opportunity to *evaluate the environment and its effect on participation*. We identified not just successes and failures of the event and the process, but of the environment as well, including physical layout challenges and distance, room layouts and food, and sup-ports present for those attending from out of town. We identi-fied environmental facilitators and barriers, and those in turn influenced the following year's event preparations. There was a consensus that midway through the process we weren't sure that we were going to pull it off, but that in the end it was a tremen-dous success. The success of the event, and the planning process lead-up, are reminders of the importance of the environment, and of the Social Imperative in supporting positive participation among individuals with aphasia.

References

Al Mahmud, A., & Martens, J. B. (2016). Social networking through email: Studying email usage patterns of persons with aphasia. *Apha-siology, 30*(2–3), 186–210.

Alary Gauvreau, C., Kairy, D., Mazer, B., Guindon, A., & Le Dorze, G. (2018). Rehabilitation strategies enhancing participation in shopping malls for persons living with a disability. *Disability and Rehabilita-tion, 40*(8), 917–925.

Antonucci, T. C., & Akiyama, H. (1987). Social networks in adult life and a preliminary examination of the convoy model. *Journal of Gerontology, 42*(5), 519–527.

Aphasia Book Connection™. (n.d.). Retrieved from http://www.apha-siacenter.net/programs/aphasia-book-club/

Beeke, S., Sirman, N., Beckley, F., Maxim, J., Edwards, S., Swinburn, K., & Best, W. (2013). *Better conversations with aphasia: An e-learning resource.* Available at https://extend.ucl.ac.uk/

Behn, N., Hilari, K., Marshall, J., Simpson, A., Northcott, S., Thomas, S., . . . McVicker, S. (2019). SUpporting Well-being Through PEeR-Befriending (SUPERB) Trial: An exploration of fidelity in peer-befriending for people with aphasia. *Brain Injury, 33*(Suppl. 1), 303–304.

Behn, N., Marshall, J., Togher, L., & Cruice, M. (2019). Feasibility and initial efficacy of project-based treatment for people with ABI. *International Journal of Language and Communication Disorders, 54*(3), 465–478.

Bernstein-Ellis, E., & Avent, J. (2013, November) *Increasing communicative access for individuals with aphasia at national parks through partnership and inclusion.* Presented at the American Speech-Language-Hearing Association Conference, Chicago, IL.

Beukelman, D. R., Hux, K., Dietz, A., McKelvey, M., & Weissling, K. (2015). Using visual scene displays as communication support options for people with chronic, severe aphasia: A summary of AAC research and future research directions. *Augmentative and Alternative Communication, 31*(3), 234–245.

Blackstone, S., & Hunt-Berg, M. (2003). *Social networks: A communication inventory for individuals with complex communication needs and their communication partners.* Verona, WI: Attainment Company.

Boles, L. (2009). *Aphasia Couples Therapy (ACT) workbook.* San Diego, CA: Plural Publishing.

Burns, M. I., Baylor, C. R., Morris, M. A., McNalley, T. E., & Yorkston, K. M. (2012). Training healthcare providers in patient–provider communication: What speech-language pathology and medical education can learn from one another. *Aphasiology, 26*(5), 673–688.

Carling-Rowland, A., Black, S., McDonald, L., & Kagan, A. (2014). Increasing access to fair capacity evaluation for discharge decision-making for people with aphasia: A randomised controlled trial. *Aphasiology, 28*(6), 750–765.

Carney, A., Elman, R., Rome, A., & Scheiner, L. (2019, March). *Creating aphasia-friendly emergency and disaster planning information.* Presentation at the Aphasia Access Leadership Summit, Baltimore, MD.

Cherney, L. R., Oehring, A. K., Whipple, K., & Rubenstein, T. (2011). "Waiting on the words": Procedures and outcomes of a drama class for individuals with aphasia. *Seminars in Speech and Language, 32*(3), 229–242.

Coles, J., & Snow, B. (2011). Applying the principles of peer mentorship in persons with aphasia. *Topics in Stroke Rehabilitation*, *18*(2), 106-111.

Cruice, M., Worrall, L., & Hickson, L. (2006). Quantifying aphasic people's social lives in the context of non-aphasic peers. *Aphasiology*, *20*(12), 1210–1225.

Csikszentmihalyi, M. (1975). *Beyond boredom and anxiety*. San Francisco, CA: Jossey-Bass.

Csikszentmihalyi, M., Abuhamdeh, S., & Nakamura, J. (2014). Flow. In M. Csikszentmihalyi (Ed.), *Flow and the foundations of positive psychology* (pp. 227–238). Dordrecht, Netherlands: Springer.

Cunningham, R., & Ward, C. (2003). Evaluation of a training programme to facilitate conversation between people with aphasia and their partners. *Aphasiology*, *17*(8), 687–707.

Delle Fave, A., & Massimini, F. (2004). Bringing subjectivity into focus: Optimal experiences, life themes, and person-centered rehabilitation. In P. A. Linley & S. Joseph (Eds.), *Positive psychology in practice* (pp. 581–597). Hoboken, NJ: Wiley.

Duchan, J., Jennings, M., Barrett, R., & Butler, B. (2006). Communication access to the arts. *Topics in Language Disorders*, *26*(3), 210–220.

Duff, M. C., Gallegos, D. R., Cohen, N. J., & Tranel, D. (2013). Learning in Alzheimer's disease is facilitated by social interaction. *Journal of Comparative Neurology*, *521*(18), 4356–4369.

Elman, R. J. (Ed.), (2007). *Group treatment of neurogenic communication disorders: The expert clinician's approach* (2nd ed.). San Diego, CA: Plural Publishing.

Elman, R. J. (2016). Aphasia centers and the life participation approach to aphasia: A paradigm change. *Topics in Language Disorders*, *36*(2), 154–167.

Garrett, K. L., & Lasker, J. P. (2005). *The Multimodal Communication Screening Test for persons with Aphasia (MCST-A)*. Retrieved from https://cehs.unl.edu/aac/aphasia-assessment-materials/

Garrett, K., & Lasker, J. (2013). Adults with severe aphasia. In D. Beukelman & P. Mirenda (Eds.), *Augmentative and alternative communication* (4th ed., pp. 405–446). London, UK: Brookes.

Government of Canada. (2019) *Accessible transportation for persons with disabilities regulations, SOR/2019-244*. Retrieved from http://gazette.gc.ca/rp-pr/p2/2019/2019-07-10/html/sor-dors244-eng.html

Haley, K. L., Cunningham, K. T., Barry, J., & de Riesthal, M. (2019). Collaborative goals for communicative life participation in aphasia: The FOURC model. *American Journal of Speech-Language Pathology*, *28*(1), 1–13.

Hawthorne, G. (2006). Measuring social isolation in older adults: Development and initial validation of the friendship scale. *Social Indicators Research*, *77*(3), 521–548.

Hengst, J. A., Duff, M. C., & Jones, T. A. (2019). Enriching communicative environments: Leveraging advances in neuroplasticity for improving outcomes in neurogenic communication disorders. *American Journal of Speech-Language Pathology*, *28*(1S), 216–229.

Henriksson, I., & Laakso, K. (2019). Book talk and aphasia: The power of a book. *International Journal of Language and Communication Disorders*. *55*(1), 136–148.

Hersh, D., Worrall, L., Howe, T., Sherratt, S., & Davidson, B. (2012). SMARTER goal setting in aphasia rehabilitation. *Aphasiology*, *26*(2), 220–233.

Ho, K. M., Weiss, S. J., Garrett, K. L., & Lloyd, L. L. (2005). The effect of remnant and pictographic books on the communicative interaction of individuals with global aphasia. *Augmentative and Alternative Communication*, *21*(3), 218–232.

Hoepner, J., Clark, M., Sather, T., & Knutson, M. (2012, September). Immersion learning at aphasia camp. *EBE Briefs: Evidence-Based Education*, pp. 1–10.

Holland, A. (2008). Concentrating on the consequences: Consequence-oriented treatment. In N. Martin, C. Thompson & L. Worrall (Eds.), *Aphasia rehabilitation: The impairment and its consequences* (pp. 31–44). San Diego, CA: Plural Publishing.

Holland, A. L., & Nelson, R. L. (2020). *Counseling in communication disorders: A wellness perspective* (3rd ed.). San Diego, CA: Plural Publishing.

Hopper, T., Holland, A., & Rewega, M. (2002). Conversational coaching: Treatment outcomes and future directions. *Aphasiology*, *16*, 745–761.

Horton, S., Lane, K., & Shiggins, C. (2016). Supporting communication for people with aphasia in stroke rehabilitation: Transfer of training in a multidisciplinary stroke team. *Aphasiology*, *30*(5), 629–656.

Howe, T. J., Worrall, L. E., & Hickson, L. M. (2008a). Interviews with people with aphasia: Environmental factors that influence their community participation. *Aphasiology*, *22*(10), 1092–1120.

Howe, T. J., Worrall, L. E., & Hickson, L. M. (2008b). Observing people with aphasia: Environmental factors that influence their community participation. *Aphasiology*, *22*(6), 618–643.

Hux, K., Buechter, M., Wallace, S., & Weissling, K. (2010). Using visual scene displays to create a shared communication space for a person with aphasia. *Aphasiology*, *24*(5), 643–660.

Jensen, L. R., Løvholt, A. P., Sørensen, I. R., Blüdnikow, A. M., Iversen, H. K., Hougaard, A., . . . Forchhammer, H. B. (2015). Implementation of supported conversation for communication between nursing staff and in-hospital patients with aphasia. *Aphasiology*, *29*(1), 57–80.

Kagan, A. (1998). Supported conversation for adults with aphasia: Methods and resources for training conversation partners. *Aphasiology*, *12*(9), 816–830.

Kagan, A., & LeBlanc, K. (2002). Motivating for infrastructure change: Toward a communicatively accessible, participation-based stroke care system for all those affected by aphasia. *Journal of Communication Disorders*, *35*(2), 153–169.

Kagan, A., Simmons-Mackie, N., Victor, J. C., Carling-Rowland, A., Hoch, J., & Huijbregts, M., (2011). *Assessment for Living with Aphasia (ALA)*. Toronto, ON: Aphasia Institute.

Kagan, A., Simmons-Mackie, N., Victor, J. C., & Chan, M. T. (2017). Communicative access measures for stroke: Development and evaluation of a quality improvement tool. *Archives of Physical Medicine and Rehabilitation*, *98*(11), 2228–2236.

Kagan, A., Winckel, J., Black, S., Felson Duchan, J., Simmons-Mackie, N., & Square, P. (2004). A set of observational measures for rating support and participation in conversation between adults with aphasia and their conversation partners. *Topics in Stroke Rehabilitation*, *11*(1), 67–83.

Kim, E. S., Ruelling, A., Garcia, J. R., & Kajner, R. (2017). A pilot study examining the impact of aphasia camp participation on quality of life for people with aphasia. *Topics in Stroke Rehabilitation*, *24*(2), 107–113.

Knollman-Porter, K., Wallace, S. E., Brown, J. A., Hux, K., Hoagland, B. L., & Ruff, D. R. (2019). Effects of written, auditory, and combined modalities on comprehension by people with aphasia. *American Journal of Speech-Language Pathology*, *28*(3), 1206–1221.

Larsson, I., & Thorén-Jönsson, A. L. (2007). The Swedish speech interpretation service: An exploratory study of a new communication support provided to people with aphasia. *Augmentative and Alternative Communication*, *23*(4), 312–322.

Lawrie, M., Hobson, T., & Tyson, S. (2007). Volunteers and the QEII District Speech Pathology Service. *ACQuiring Knowledge in Speech, Language, and Hearing*, *9*(2), 64–67.

Lock, S., Wilkinson, R., & Bryan, K. (2001). *Supporting Partners of People with Aphasia in Relationships and Conversation (SPAARC) Assessment*. Milton Keynes, UK: Speechmark.

LPAA Project Group (Chapey, R., Duchan, J. F., Elman, R. J., Garcia, L. J., Kagan, A., Lyon, J. G., & Simmons Mackie, N.). (2000). Life participation approach to aphasia: A statement of values for the future. *The ASHA Leader, 5*(3), 4–6.

Lubinski, R. (2011). Creating a positive communication environment in long-term care. In P. Backhaus (Ed.), *Communication in elderly care: Cross-cultural perspectives* (pp. 40–61). London, UK: Continuum International.

Lyon, J. G., Cariski, D., Keisler, L., Rosenbek, J., Levine, R., Kumpula, J., . . . Blanc, M. (1997). Communication partners: Enhancing participation in life and communication for adults with aphasia in natural settings. *Aphasiology, 11*(7), 693–708.

Manning, M., MacFarlane, A., Hickey, A., & Franklin, S. (2019). Perspectives of people with aphasia post-stroke towards personal recovery and living successfully: A systematic review and thematic synthesis. *PloS One, 14*(3), e0214200.

Martin, N., Thompson, C. K., & Worrall, L. (2007). *Aphasia rehabilitation: The impairment and its consequences.* San Diego, CA: Plural Publishing.

McGilton, K., Sorin-Peters, R., Sidani, S., Rochon, E., Boscart, V., & Fox, M. (2011). Focus on communication: Increasing the opportunity for successful staff–patient interactions. *International Journal of Older People Nursing, 6*(1), 13–24.

Northcott, S., & Hilari, K. (2013). Stroke Social Network Scale: Development and psychometric evaluation of a new patient-reported measure. *Clinical Rehabilitation, 27*(9), 823–833.

O'Halloran, R., Carragher, M., & Foster, A. (2017). The consequences of the consequences: The impact of the environment on people with aphasia over time. *Topics in Language Disorders, 37*(1), 85.

O'Halloran, R., Lee, Y. S., Rose, M., & Liamputtong, P. (2014). Creating communicatively accessible healthcare environments: Perceptions of speech-language pathologists. *International Journal of Speech-Language Pathology, 16*(6), 603–614.

O'Halloran, R., Worrall, L., Toffolo, D., & Code, C. (2020). IFCI–Environment questionnaires. In *Inpatient Functional Communication Interview: Screening, assessment, and intervention* (pp. 63–68). San Diego, CA: Plural Publishing.

Page, C. G., & Rowles, G. D. (2016). "It doesn't require much effort once you get to know them": Certified nursing assistants' views of communication in long-term care. *Journal of Gerontological Nursing, 42*(4), 42–51.

Plourde, J. M., Purdy, S. C., Moore, C., Friary, P., Brown, R., & McCann, C. M. (2019). Gavel Club for people with aphasia: Communication confidence and quality of communication life. *Aphasiology, 33*(1), 73–93.

Rautakoski, P. (2014). Communication style before and after aphasia: A study among Finnish population. *Aphasiology*, 28(3), 359–376.

Rohde, A., Townley-O'Neill, K., Trendall, K., Worrall, L., & Cornwell, P. (2012). A comparison of client and therapist goals for people with aphasia: A qualitative exploratory study. *Aphasiology, 26*(10), 1298–1315.

Rose, T. A., Worrall, L. E., Hickson, L. M., & Hoffmann, T. C. (2011). Aphasia friendly written health information: Content and design characteristics. *International Journal of Speech-Language Pathology, 13*(4), 335–347

Saldert, C., Jensen, L. R., Blom Johansson, M., & Simmons-Mackie, N. (2018). Complexity in measuring outcomes after communication partner training: Alignment between goals of intervention and methods of evaluation. *Aphasiology, 32*(10), 1167–1193.

Sather, T. W., Howe, T., Nelson, N. W., & Lagerwey, M. (2017). Optimizing the experience of flow for adults with aphasia. *Topics in Language Disorders, 37*(1), 25–37.

Silverman, M. E. (2011). Community: The key to building and extending engagement for individuals with aphasia. *Seminars in Speech and Language, 32*(3), 256–267.

Simmons-Mackie N. (2008). Social approaches to aphasia intervention. In R. Chapey (Ed.), *Language intervention strategies in aphasia and related neurogenic communication disorders* (5th ed., pp. 290–318). Baltimore, MD: Lippincott Williams & Wilkins.

Simmons-Mackie, N. N., & Damico, J. S. (1996). Accounting for handicaps in aphasia: Communicative assessment from an authentic social perspective. *Disability and Rehabilitation, 18*(11), 540–549.

Simmons-Mackie, N., Elman, R. J., Holland, A. L., & Damico, J. S. (2007). Management of discourse in group therapy for aphasia. *Topics in Language Disorders, 27*(1), 5–23.

Simmons-Mackie, N., & Holland, A. L. (2011). Aphasia centers in North America: A survey. *Seminars in Speech and Language, 32*(3), 203–215.

Simmons-Mackie, N., King, J. M., & Beukelman, D. R. (Eds.). (2013). *Supporting communication for adults with acute and chronic aphasia*. Baltimore, MD: Brookes.

Simmons-Mackie, N., Raymer, A., & Cherney, L. R. (2016). Communication partner training in aphasia: An updated systematic review. *Archives of Physical Medicine and Rehabilitation, 97*(12), 2202–2221.

Solarsh, B., & Johnson, H. (2017). Developing communication access standards to maximize community inclusion for people with communication support needs. *Topics in Language Disorders*, *37*(1), 52–66.

Tarrant, M., Warmoth, K., Code, C., Dean, S., Goodwin, V. A., Stein, K., & Sugavanam, T. (2016). Creating psychological connections between intervention recipients: Development and focus group evaluation of a group singing session for people with aphasia. *BMJ Open*, *6*(2), e009652.

Thomas, S. A., Coates, E., das Nair, R., Lincoln, N. B., Cooper, C., Palmer, R., . . . Chater, T. (2016). Behavioural Activation Therapy for Depression after Stroke (BEADS): A study protocol for a feasibility randomised controlled pilot trial of a psychological intervention for post-stroke depression. *Pilot and Feasibility Studies*, *2*(1), 45.

Threats, T. (2000). The World Health Organization's revised classification: What does it mean for speech-language pathology? *Journal of Medical Speech Language Pathology, 8*(3), xiii–xviii.

Tregea, S., & Brown, K. (2013). What makes a successful peer-led aphasia support group? *Aphasiology*, *27*(5), 581–598.

Walker, J. P., & Jacques, K. (2016, October). *Speech therapy in a virtual world: Building friendships in a telepractice aphasia communication group*. Poster presented at the 54th Annual Academy of Aphasia Meeting, Llandudno, UK. In *Frontiers in Psychology Conference Abstract: 54th Annual Academy of Aphasia Meeting*. https://doi.org/10.3389/conf.fpsyg.2016.68.00013

Wielaert, S., van de Sandt-Koenderman, M. W., Dammers, N., & Sage, K. (2018). ImPACT: A multifaceted implementation for conversation partner training in aphasia in Dutch rehabilitation settings. *Disability and Rehabilitation, 40*(1), 76–89.

Woolf, S., & Aron, L. (2013). *U.S. health in international perspective: Shorter lives, poorer health*. Washington, DC: National Research Council and Committee on Population—National Academies Press.

World Health Organization. (2001). *International classification of functioning, disability and health: ICF*. Geneva, Switzerland: Author.

5

STORIES AT THE HEART OF LIFE PARTICIPATION

BOTH THE TELLING AND LISTENING MATTER

Katie A. Strong and Barbara B. Shadden

To give the gift of listening is to appreciate receiving the gift of a story. Not just understanding this reciprocity but embracing it seems to me to be the beginning of clinical work.

—Frank, 2007, p. 25

The Social Imperative for Supporting Story Therapeutically

When we say stories are at the heart of life participation, what we mean is that we are the stories we tell. Our stories allow us to frame our sense of identity or self, in part because stories are at the heart of our interactions as humans. All of us, whether we have aphasia or not, process life through stories, particularly significant life events. As we process those events, our stories change based on how we feel about those events and about ourselves. Who we choose to share our stories with, and how they react to them, affects how we feel about ourselves, and how and if we will choose to share that story again in the future.

The Life Participation Approach to Aphasia (LPAA) has been transformative in how we as speech-language pathologists (SLPs) approach our work with individuals affected by aphasia. By suggesting that life participation should be a primary intervention goal, LPAA challenges us to focus on " . . . the dual function of communication—transmitting and receiving messages and establishing and maintaining meaningful social links" (LPAA Project Group, 2000, p. 2). We believe that both the telling (transmitting) and receiving (listening) of stories fit this dual function of communication. Further, at the heart of LPAA is a fundamental understanding of the social impact of aphasia and the centrality of social interactions and experiences to life participation. Stories allow us to connect with others and maintain meaningful social experiences and relationships. We feel strongly that supporting individuals living with aphasia through the listening and telling of stories is a part of the social imperative that is the foundation of this book.

Traditionally, as SLPs, we think of intervention as either restorative or compensatory. Restorative therapy techniques target repairing and rebuilding damaged neural networks, whereas compensatory therapy techniques target the use of adaptive tools and behaviors. We would like to add the concept of transformative interventions as another approach. Just as LPAA has been transformative in how we view our work, we believe that using stories therapeutically has transformative power. Used purposefully, stories have the potential to change us by linking the past, present, and future in a meaningful way. In addition, these changes can impact life participation and well-being.

The Negative Impact of Aphasia on Health and Quality of Life

Aphasia has a significant negative impact on health and quality of life (QoL) outcomes. In fact, secondary consequences of aphasia include higher disability risk than stroke without aphasia, depression, social isolation and loneliness, negative impact on identity and on communicative engagement, and sense of help-lessness (Simmons-Mackie, 2018). If that isn't enough, people with aphasia report loss of friends, strain on family, and reduced social activity (Northcott, Moss, Harrison, & Hilari, 2015). Loss of friends is associated with loneliness and social isolation, leading to additional negative health impacts (World Health Organization, 2003).

One way we as humans connect with friends and family is through story, which relies heavily on language. For example, telling someone a story about your day, sharing about a time when . . . , or expanding on a conversation about a common experience are all ways in which we connect with others on a daily basis. People with aphasia are disadvantaged at sharing these seemingly small stories that make a large contribution to our relationships. Disrupted social interactions can also impact self-esteem and identity adversely (Shadden & Koski, 2007). A person's primary tool for story navigation is language, the very tool that aphasia has damaged (Shadden & Koski, 2007).

Far Reaching Impact of Aphasia on Friends and Family

The reach of aphasia extends to friends and family members. Living with aphasia in the family can increase loneliness, burden of responsibility due to role changes, and loss of friends by family members (Natterlund, 2010). Communication in the family may deteriorate due to aphasia (LeDorze, Tremblay, & Croteau, 2009). Although family members are not typically included directly in therapy (Hallé, LeDorze, & Mingant, 2014) they have expressed interest in being more included in order to learn communication strategies, care for their own well-being, and manage new responsibilities (Howe et al., 2012). In other words, friends and family members have their own stories to explore and tell and for us as clinicians to hear.

A Call for Action: Transformation Through Story

As aphasia is a chronic health condition, providing supports and intervention that address domains beyond language impairment is crucial. In her report on the *State of Aphasia in North America*, Simmons-Mackie (2018) invites stakeholders interested in the future of aphasia services to join her in a call to action to transform the lives of people affected by aphasia. One way SLPs can respond to this social imperative is by better supporting those living with aphasia in their use of stories. All stories matter. Small stories allow us allow us to engage in everyday happenings and acts of self-presentation and validation and big stories provide an opportunity provide an opportunity to reflect on life. Stories honor identities of the past, reconstruct current identities with aphasia, and imagine a future filled with hope in living successfully with aphasia.

In this chapter, we expand on the concept of story, its relationship to identity, and how it is at the heart of life participation. Next, we explore the fundamentals of listening, an essential ingredient in story exchange. We end the chapter with a discussion of strategies SLPs can use in supporting the telling of stories in therapeutic environments, including recent evidence-based approaches. We hope you will agree that sharing one's stories is at the heart of living successfully with aphasia and is a valuable therapeutic target.

Stories at the Heart of Human Interaction and Life Participation

"Storytelling is in our blood. We are the storytelling species" (Atkinson, 2002, p. 122). In fact, storytelling has been a defining attribute of humankind since homo sapiens first appeared.

With the evolving ability to understand and use language, stories emerged (Harari, 2015). Stories became tools to share experiences necessary for survival, then expanded to be part of humans' attempts to explain the world around them. As Atkinson (2002) suggests, "In traditional communities of the past, stories played a central role in the lives of the people . . . Stories told from generation to generation carried enduring values as well as lessons about life lived deeply" (p. 121).

The sharing of daily experiences and of past history through story also provided the earliest mechanisms to begin to codify a sense of self and identity—for the individual and for those around him or her. Story exchange anchored social interactions and allowed us to evolve socially. So, language, story, and identity have been inextricably linked through centuries.

Story may mean different things to different people in different contexts. For some, story may be a series of family accounts passed down through the generations to explain the family's roots in Finland or the success story of a great-grandparent. For others, story evokes one's life story or autobiography. Some stories are fictional, as in fairy tales, but also universal in a given culture. For example, English speakers may think of Cinderella or Jack and the Beanstalk.

Yet stories can be, and often are, less formal, more immediate, and seemingly mundane. Often these types of stories are referred to as everyday personal narratives. They may be conversational anecdotes of something recent that has happened, such as a humorous retelling of a first date disaster the night before. They may also be sharing an experience from years earlier that had an impact on one's life direction or purpose. A personal narrative may relate to some aspect of who we feel we are, or want to be seen as in a certain situation or with certain individuals. Regardless of type of story, each is an integral part of everyday life.

In speech-language pathology, story and narrative also evoke multiple perspectives. Traditionally, these terms bring to mind picture description, story re-tell, monologues, and related discourse tasks. As SLPs, we often listen for cohesive stories that have a beginning, middle, and an end, and then evaluate the structure and quality of a story based on various aspects such as grammar, word choice, sequencing, and so forth. In this chapter, however, we are exploring the life function of narrative, particularly as related to identity work. Hyden (2008) suggests that we should conceptualize story and storytelling as social action, through which " . . . social states are . . . established, negotiated, and changed" (p. 48).

We encourage you to examine story with a broader lens in working with people living with aphasia. This lens focuses in on the power of story to influence how people view themselves and understand significant life events, including moving forward from such events. In our field, texts by Hinckley (2007) and Shadden, Hagstrom, and Koski (2008) provided a preliminary platform for SLPs to explore this expanded view of narrative. Part of understanding story involves understanding its links to identity and the process of social construction that connects the two.

Story, Identity, and Social Construction: We are the Stories We Tell

Taylor (1994) defines identity quite simply as "who we are, where we've been, and where we are going" (p. 33). Our view of who we are is heavily influenced by our life experiences and how we choose to portray these experiences through story. So, stories are reflections of our selves. When we engage in storytelling, we are actually providing the listener with guidance about how we want to be understood (Bamberg, 2012). McAdams (2008) uses the term narrative identity to link identity and story and to underscore the timeline of identity. In 2018, McAdams stated, "Narrative identity is a special kind of story—a story about how I came to be the person I am becoming" (p. 364). He proposes that, if we listen to how a story is told, we can learn about how others view themselves. In turn, if we listen to our own stories, we can learn about how we view ourselves.

Story exchange is a fundamentally social act, and the term co-construction is used frequently to capture the role the listener plays in this process. Stories need an audience in order to have a life. We are selective in choosing stories to share depending on our social partner, the setting, and the broader culture. Very few of us would choose to tell the same story anecdotes to a parent, a teacher, a first date, or a new group of coworkers. One reason stories vary is because they are integral to forming relationships and to acceptance in a group or organization.

Stories are a way to make meaning out of events that happen to us. For example, you probably have a story about how you came to become an SLP. You may also have a story about the birth of your child, or another significant milestone, or perhaps a negative experience, such as the time you were betrayed by a friend or colleague. Over time, through the telling and retelling and listener responses, these stories may evolve. Throughout, language is the essential tool that is used to develop and share stories.

Impact of Aphasia on Story and Identity

This same language tool for meaning-making and identity framing is damaged directly by aphasia. Ironically, having a stroke and subsequent aphasia is the kind of major life event that requires active sense-making and that fractures the continuity of the life story and one's identity. Imagine having a near death experience, perhaps no longer able to work, and then not being able to communicate with others to share your basic needs let along your hopes and dreams. These challenges are at the core of the profound psychosocial consequences of living with aphasia. People with aphasia need support in accessing their language tool in order to develop and share both small and big stories. SLPs are well suited to provide needed language and communicative support, but to play such a role, SLPs need an understanding of the nature and range of story types we all produce in our lives.

Types of Stories, Small and Big

There are probably as many different definitions of "story" as there are types of stories. Of course, narrative can be analyzed for specific elements such as language structure and organization of information. However, our focus is more on the content of and reason for the telling of a story. It may be helpful to consider the idea of small (little) and big personal stories (Bamberg, 2012;

McAdams, 2018) to characterize human storytelling, as described by Strong and Shadden (2020).

Small Stories: Everyday Personal Narratives

Bamberg (2010) suggests small stories most frequently play a role in relationships and social interactions, where we seek validation. The term "everyday personal narratives" or personal stories are used interchangeably with the small stories. As defined in the Linguistic Underpinnings of Narrative in Aphasia (LUNA) project (Dipper & Cruice, 2018), these stories tend to be short anecdotes of events that the speaker has been part of, or that have been witnessed or told by others. Small stories may be as brief as a personal observation injected into a conversation. They may also be the sharing of an experience from years earlier that had an impact on the speaker's life direction or purpose. As personal stories, they often relate to some aspect of who we feel we are or want others to see in us.

Everyday personal narratives often occur in informal conversational exchanges. Bamberg (2012) emphasizes the fact that these conversations are in fact forums for self-narration and require give-and-take between conversational partners, a premise echoed by Holstein and Gubrium (2000) who suggest that small stories provide ongoing opportunities for restorying one's life and self every day. Personal narratives reflect conscious or unconscious choices we make as to what to share with whom under what circumstances.

Think about what any of us typically chooses to share about our life and experiences when we meet new people or are placed in a new environment. Most of us are selective in choosing stories based on the listener and circumstances, or even in selecting personal elements to inject into an ongoing conversation. Now imagine the loss in spontaneity and self-disclosure when aphasia disrupts the language tool.

The everyday personal narrative tends to be relatively brief and restricted in content, scope, and place in life trajectory. The speaker may or may not include reflection on the story, although small stories often provide opportunities for reframing self. If a story is quite specific to life events and experiences, McAdams

(2018) suggests we might view them as parts of an anthology of stories by a single author. As such, they become an important part of the bigger life story.

Big Stories: Illness Narratives and Life Story/Autobiography

Illness narratives are one example of specialized stories that are invariably situated in the context of the life trajectory. Bamberg (2012) would consider them a type of big story in that they address a complicating or meaningful life event. Whole texts have been written on the topic of illness narratives (most recently, Lucius-Hoene, Homberg, & Myer, 2018). An illness narrative is what we tell when we attempt to make sense of a major health crisis by creating a new story around this crisis and trying to use that story to explain what happened, what is going on now, and potentially how we move forward. Illness narrative formulation can be an act of sense-making and incorporating illness events into the broader life story (Hyden, 1997). Sharing an illness narrative gives others a chance to comment and to demonstrate recognition, acceptance, and participation in reconstructing life stories. In other words, the social sharing is crucial; it allows for buy-in to the illness story.

Within aphasiology, a number of researchers have elicited and examined closely stroke or aphasia narratives, often focusing on the more structural or linguistic aspects of narrative (e.g., Ulatowska et al., 2013). More recently, research has established that non-guided illness narratives can be effective in identifying thematic areas important to people with stroke and aphasia (Pluta, Ulatowska, Gawron, Sobanska, & Lojek, 2014).

Frank (2013) talks about three major illness narrative frames that are commonly cited. These include: (1) the restitution story, (2) the chaos story, and (3) the quest story. A narrative of restitution tells a story of life as usual, being disrupted by illness, and then being restored to the previous life. In the case of having a stroke and aphasia, a restitution narrative might be something like, "I had a stroke and aphasia and I recovered from it fully. I'm now back at work and living life as I always had." According to Frank, restitution narratives are what we want to hear.

Life was great, tragedy happened, and now my life is restored. Given the chronicity of aphasia, restitution narratives may occur infrequently in the stories of the clients on a typical speech therapy caseload.

In contrast, chaos narratives are difficult to hear. The chaos story, often found in instances of profound illness or disability, is a vicious cycle of falling apart. Problems seem unending and will probably get worse but certainly cannot be treated. Listeners can be overwhelmed by chaos stories—the lack of feasible action is difficult to manage, and the story does not really have the usual narrative beginning, middle, and end. Chaos stories can project a sense of hopelessness. Finally, the quest story frames an illness when the condition itself may not be fixable but there is still insight to be gained. Illness is viewed as a journey. A quest narrative of a person with aphasia may include advocating for awareness of aphasia or sharing with others how that person has changed for the better from the experience of having aphasia.

Frank (2013) developed this narrative framework to provide health care providers with a starting point from which to listen to and support clients who are sharing experiences about their illness. Illness narrative types are not intended to be tools for categorizing clients. Instead, they reflect the fact that " . . . people tell the stories they need to tell in order to work through the situation in which they find themselves" (Frank, 2007, p. 34).

The field of narrative medicine has targeted the shift to a focus on patient stories as a way of capturing and validating the unique lived experience of illness and the changing relationships between health care providers and patients (Charon & Montello, 2002). Narrative perspectives have influenced other disciplines as well as medicine. In most instances, big stories have received the most focus, often in the form of a life story or autobiography.

Whereas most of us share bits and pieces of our life story in daily interactions, it is less common to engage in the process of framing the story of our expanded life trajectory. If we look at people with aphasia and their life participation needs, it is fairly obvious that their experienced life changes, identity challenges, and the break in continuity of life story make them obvious targets for life story interventions. The challenge is that humans do not automatically know how to tell their life story. We all require guidance in this process. And although the creation and sharing of life stories may be critical for many individuals facing major life changes, the unique challenge presented by aphasia is its impact on the language tool that is at the heart of framing and communicating parts of one's life story. That is where SLPs may bring a unique skill set to the process. Helping a client generate and then tell his or her story would appear to be a reasonable goal in intervention for those living with aphasia and seeking full life participation.

There are a number of tools and approaches from other disciplines available for life story or autobiographic work, both with individuals and groups. In gerontology, exploration of narratives of aging have shed light on the experience of aging individuals in our society (Bruner, 1999; Randall & Kenyon, 2000). Reminiscence and life story review have been identified as powerful tools in healthy adaptation to aging and in well-being (Kenyon, 2003), as well as useful approaches for adults with neurological impairments (Harris, 1997). Autobiography has received renewed attention (e.g., Birren & Cochran, 2001). In the field of psychology, the importance of the construct of life story has emerged (McAdams, 2008), and narrative intervention has also become more prevalent in practice. There are emerging models for types of life story interventions for a variety of clinical populations, including persons with stroke and aphasia. Examples of these are provided in the next section of this chapter.

Incorporating Story into Your LPAA Practice—What the SLP Can Do

Gubrium and Holstein (1998) " . . . use the term 'narrative practice' to characterize simultaneously the activities of storytelling, the resources used to tell stories, and the auspices under which stories are told" (p. 164). As SLPs who embrace the LPAA approach, we may also want to consider our clinical work to be a kind of narrative practice. So, what does that mean? As will be discussed, one major role of the SLP is to serve as an active listener and conversational partner, not just a health care provider focusing on the client's ability to convey desired language content. We need to set the stage for story generation. We need to receive and support stories in the context of our relationship with a client or family members. For our clients to move forward in life, and make sense of what has happened and changed for them, congruence between one's old and new stories and the perceptions of others is essential.

It Starts with Listening

Regardless of small or big story, a story needs a listener. As SLPs, we know the value of listening to our clients and their families. However, we may not fully recognize the extent of power that listening really has on a story and in turn identity. Therefore, in this chapter we have intentionally front-loaded the topic of listening before addressing the telling side of storytelling. Truly listening—and acknowledging what you have heard—is potentially one of the most powerful tools a clinician has.

Most of us have had the experience of having a client tell us a story during a session. Perhaps we've heard a particular story many times before. The story may take some time to tell. And, we may have felt that the story, "while nice to hear, wasn't a part of the session." Or if we were honest, maybe we thought to ourselves, "Oh here it comes again. Do I have to hear this story one more time?" As clinicians, we are goal focused with our clients. We have a carefully scheduled plan for each session. The demands of providing reimbursable services are real. So are the constraints of busy schedules. However, we also need to be available to hear stories that clients feel they need to tell us. Frank (2007) provides perspective that as long as a story continues to be told, the work of that situation needs navigating. And although we as clinicians may occasionally find this telling and retelling frustrating, listening to stories signals the person with aphasia that they are not alone and validates that what they have to say is important.

Listening is an essential ingredient in storytelling. How a story is received influences how that story is told. Think about a time in your life when you were telling a story and you felt like the person you were telling your story to wasn't listening. Or that the person didn't really hear the message you were sharing. Did you feel compelled to continue sharing information? Probably not. Chances are you changed what you were sharing or stopped sharing altogether. In this instance, the listener negatively influenced your story. Now switch gears and think about a time you felt 'heard' when telling story. The person you were communicating with truly was present and listened to your story. How did you feel? How did this feeling differ from the first example? What are some of the traits that the listener exhibited that made you feel 'heard'? Now think about a recent therapy session you had with a client or a family member who shared a story with you. Did you respond to them as a person, or as a clinician? Was your focus on the language and effectiveness in framing the story, or on the person's experience?

We ask you to explore this because the relationship between someone telling a story and their listener is important. In fact, the relationship between the storyteller and listener is more influential than the actual content that is shared. Stories are told to cultivate relationships (Frank, 2007). If we only listen for certain types of stories, Frank warns us we may limit the relationship with the person who is telling us that story. We need to be open to receiving and listening to the stories our clients and their families are telling us. Because stories are socially coconstructed (Hyden, 2008), you, as a listener, are essentially a collaborator or conarrator of a story (Randall, Prior, & Skaborn, 2006). No two listeners are alike, and a relationship is created between the storyteller and listener which impacts what gets told and how it is told (Randall et al., 2006).

Worrall and colleagues (2010) have provided evidence that relationship-centered care (RCC) is fundamental to aphasia rehabilitation. If you think about it, that really makes sense. RCC is defined as care in which all participants appreciate the importance of their relationships with one another (Beach, Inui, & the Relationship-Centered Care Network, 2006). In the case of aphasia rehabilitation, participants include the person with aphasia, family members, or other stakeholders close that person, and the clinician. Beach and colleagues (2006) suggest that the principles of RCC encourage us to not only acknowledge but also embrace "who a person is" or the identity of participants, including the clinician. In the relationship, what is told is influenced by perceptions of both the listener and the teller about each other. All of these factors are fluid during the actual telling of a story.

Listening to stories serves other functions as well. Authentic listening can assist in increasing communication between health care providers and patients and also identify important topics and needs of patients in order to provide meaningful intervention (Pluta et al., 2014). Hersh (2015) argues that when health care providers listen to the stories of their clients, particularly those with moderate to severe aphasia, they are giving a voice not only to their experiences with biographic disruption, such as living with stroke and aphasia, but also allowing their opinion to be heard in providing feedback on the services they receive throughout their rehabilitation journey.

Much of what has been discussed in this section can and should be considered best practices in counseling. In their text on a wellness perspective on counseling, Holland and Nelson (2018) provide excellent insight into listening and understanding as a "quiet" skill essential for counseling clients with communication disorders. Practical information accompanies listening exercises in this resource.

One major caution before moving on to the telling of stories: Frank (2007) warns us that there is always the danger of a health care provider taking on listening as a routine task. If listening, and narrative elicitation, become clinical techniques that are simply part of a checklist of items to cover, the uniqueness of truly listening and truly being heard is virtually eliminated. The power of story will be diminished.

Ways SLPs Can Support the Telling of Stories

Obviously, the listening to and telling of stories are interrelated. The focus now shifts to ways you may support the expression of both small and big stories in your therapy sessions and even consider some more structured life story work based on the aphasiology research to date. There is "no one size fits all" for supporting stories clinically.

It is beneficial to distinguish the product (the actual story told) from the process (the experience of telling the story). The product, though important, is not as potentially transformative as the process of sharing a personal story. The process depends in part on the clinician's approach to encouraging story, captured in the idea and acronym of taking the PULSE of the client and others living with aphasia (Figure 5–1). PULSE stands for Partnerships, Uniqueness, Listening, Supporting Stories of Self, and Exploring Life with Aphasia.

The PULSE acronym was originally developed to help SLPs engage in supporting identity work and life participation through story with their clients with aphasia. An expanded explanation of PULSE can be found in Strong and Shadden (2020). A central component to PULSE is listening, which we have already addressed.

Knowing different methods and clinical skills to apply when helping your clients engage in sharing stories helps you to be more open to the opportunities for storying that present themselves. In one survey, SLPs reported believing story and identity work were important but did not regularly use story therapeutically to support identity reconstruction in their clients with aphasia (Strong & Nelson, 2012). Many SLPs do not feel comfortable with doing this work this as it is an expansion of

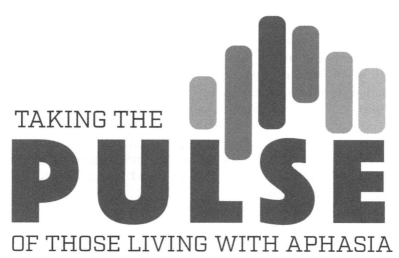

Figure 5–1. Taking the PULSE of those living with aphasia. Copyright Shadden and Strong, 2020.

the traditional use of story in speech-language pathology (e.g., story re-tell, discourse analysis, etc.). Evidence-based methods for coconstructing small and big stories that support identity and well-being are emerging in the current literature in aphasiology and are discussed below.

Ways to Support Everyday Small Stories

Taking the PULSE of our clients can be particularly effective in encouraging the small personal everyday stories. It is often those small stories that provide the foundation for relationship-building and identity renegotiation. People with aphasia and their significant others often report missing these kinds of inter-actions in their lives most. From the moment a client enters the therapy room or the group treatment setting, if SLPs present themselves as truly listening to the small stories and uses the PULSE elements to set up an environment welcoming to the exchange of small stories, it is more likely that the person with aphasia will want to share personal narratives.

One recent approach to supporting small stories in a more structured manner can be found in the LUNA project introduced earlier (Dipper & Cruice, 2018). LUNA uses everyday personal narratives to support real-life communication by targeting stories that are of importance to the person with aphasia, thus target-ing identity and at the same time target language production at the word, sentence, and discourse levels. LUNA incorporates evidence-based methods such as semantic-feature analysis and mapping theory, paired with personal storytelling. LUNA is a four-phase research program that is currently underway. Pre-liminary results are promising in providing evidence for gains in both functional communication goals and improved psycho-social well-being. More information on LUNA can be found at https://blogs.city.ac.uk/luna/

Ways to Support Illness Narratives and Big Stories

We've talked about illness narratives and big stories previ-ously. Now we apply them directly to working with people with aphasia. Within the aphasia literature, many interventions inte-grate illness narratives into big stories about life. This makes sense, as stroke and aphasia are a major biographic disruption that can benefit from navigating life changes.

In the Life Thread Model, Ellis-Hill, Payne, and Ward (2008) have applied the concept of narratives to reformulating identity and continuity in life story with individuals with stroke. This model uses a metaphor where stories represent strands of ourselves that are created and recreated throughout life. Strands of the thread can be frayed or broken by life events, such as the disruption caused by stroke and aphasia. Strands can also be rewoven into a stronger thread. The essence of this model is how clinicians can support a positive sense of self through the creation of narratives that are about learning how to live a life that is not dominated by stroke or aphasia. Although the Life Threads Model is theoretical in nature, one practical tool available for clinicians to utilize is the Guided Autobiography tool created by McAdams (1997) and available from the Northwestern University Foley Center for the Study of Lives. This tool is an exercise exploring eight different types of events that clinicians could use themselves to explore their own life stories, or to use with their clients. The Guided Autobiography tool can be accessed at https://www.sesp.northwestern.edu/foley/instruments/guided/

Interventions from other disciplines have been adapted to support individuals with aphasia in exploring big stories. Specifically, from narrative gerontology, guided autobiography (GAB; Birren & Cochran, 2001) is a method of exploring life events through writing and sharing within a group. GAB been adapted for persons with stroke (Keegan, 2013) and for persons with aphasia (Richman & Hartman, 2013). Through GAB, life with stroke and aphasia is explored through six themes ranging from "Life Before Your Stroke," to "Inventing a New Normal," to "What's Next for You?" Similarly, from the field of social work, guided-self-determination (GSD) is a method in which storytelling through a combination of individual and group sessions to target positive identity and well-being. GSD has been adapted for persons with stroke and aphasia (Bronken, Kirkevold, Martinsen, & Kvinge, 2012). The biographic-narrative approach combines individual interviews with group therapy to target improved health outcomes for people with aphasia through individual and group intervention (Corsten, Schimpf, Konradi, Keilmann, & Hardering, 2015). This approach has been identified as a lower level intensity psychological intervention in stepped care that SLPs are well suited to provide (Ryan et al., 2020). Another approach, the "My Story" Project, was developed by the first author of this chapter as a means to provide clinicians with a practical tool to use in supporting clients with aphasia in exploring life with aphasia through the process of creating a story targeting aspects of "Who I was before my aphasia, My stroke and aphasia, and My future" (Strong, 2015). Outcomes from storytellers with aphasia who participated in this project reported themes of "More than a story: My life came back to life" indicating the positive emotional experience it was to co-construct a story about their life (Strong, Lagerwey, & Shadden, 2018). Each of these interventions intentionally weaves together illness narratives and big stories to support the integration of aphasia into a more positive identity.

Groups have a powerful place for the telling of stories for people with aphasia. In fact, being able to share some of one's illness experience with others with similar experiences can provide a powerful sense of support and community. We all know the value of being able to identify with a broader group of people who have walked in our shoes and who understand us through their own personal experiences. Most therapeutic or support groups provide these opportunities to share common ground through personal story (Rappaport, 1993). Participation in groups that offer opportunities to share stroke/aphasia experiences provides people with an opportunity to develop a sense of belonging and regain a sense of self-worth and responsibility for their own life while shedding the negative perception of "stroke victim" (Lund, Melhus, & Sveen, 2017; Shadden & Agan, 2004; Shadden, 2007). Elman (2007) and Simmons-Mackie and Elman (2011) provide excellent resources for group intervention for persons with aphasia.

Some stories need additional supports from mental health professionals who are better equipped to address stories of healing. Considering referral to such resources is important. Offering to collaborate with colleagues in the counseling professions, to provide the communicative support needed for those with aphasia, is yet another vehicle for SLPs to support life participation processes (Ryan et al., 2020).

We hope this introduction will spark your interest in supporting your clients who are interested in using story to explore their identity and well-being. We also anticipate that this area of the field will continue to develop and hope that interventions for both big and small stories continue to develop and expand into practical tools and approaches that clinicians can use with their clients in supporting successful life with aphasia.

Supporting the Stories of Family and Friends

Aphasia has long been described as a family illness (Buck, 1963) because the language impairment affects everyone's communication, not just that of the person with aphasia. Life changes and losses can be experienced by spouses, parents, siblings, and extended family members, as well as friends. All of these individuals share the same core human drive as the person with aphasia to process life change through stories, small and/or big. Most, if not all, experience shifts in their sense of who they are, as their life trajectory after stroke and aphasia become part of their lives. The need for validation of identity is ongoing.

Just like the person with aphasia, family members and friends have a story to process and tell (Frank, 2007). Often, they choose to share their story, or parts of it, with us as SLPs. Sometimes we are open to this, but other times we may not recognize the importance of these stories for healing. Listening to stories of friends and families can be tricky. Time constraints from busy clinic caseloads and reimbursement pressure impacts being open to receive such stories. As SLPs, we may feel that a family or friend's story isn't directly related to the goals or plan of care for our client. These challenges and preconceptions may lead us to directly or inadvertently shut down family and friends from sharing their stories.

The second author of this chapter has lived both sides of this reality—an SLP for many years working with those with aphasia, and then the spouse of a stroke survivor who acquired aphasia. For over a decade, she had led a stroke support group, made up primarily of couples living with aphasia. After her husband's stroke, when the support group resumed, she returned to spending the second half of each session with the spouses. Before her husband's stroke, the narrative in the spouse breakout group was one of mutual support, with a strong focus on the story of the stroke survivor. After the second author became a true "member" of the spouse group, the narrative shifted dramatically to a focus on stories of the spouses' challenges and stresses including some pretty tough feelings about the path their lives had taken. The only change? Presumably the fact that the spouses may have finally felt that the SLP could understand their stories. The take home message? As SLPs, we need to be as honest and open to hearing the authentic stories, big and small, of those seeking to participate fully in life with aphasia.

We encourage you to consider how to support the exploration of stories with families and friends within and beyond the walls (or confines) of therapy sessions. Being open to receiving these stories is a first step. Once again, listening plays a major role in receiving such stories. Sometimes family and friends just need to be heard. This does not always take significant amounts of time.

Conclusions

In 2007, Shadden and Hagstrom stated that:

At its core, the premise of life participation as a primary intervention goal must encompass the role of communication in renegotiating a sense of self or identity. Life participation must address more than engagement in desired activities. It must target an individual's ability to participate in core social interactions that allow narrative exploration of one's life story and associated sense of self or identity. In effect, it must actively support the biographical accommodation needed to maintain a sense of a meaningful lifeline (p. 330).

More than a decade later, this statement of social imperative remains relevant. Narrative is indeed one of the most fundamental life concerns of humans, not in the restricted sense of telling a story with good organization, but more broadly, in terms of framing and supporting one's life story and identity.

Questions remain about the role of relationships in the treatment paradigm, as well as the degree of personal engagement or disengagement appropriate for the clinician. It is our premise that SLPs are uniquely posed to understand and support the stories of life with aphasia, and in doing so, facilitate fuller life participation with aphasia. Clinicians can choose to focus primarily on providing an environment for sharing everyday personal narratives, or more purposefully, they can elicit and support illness narratives or create more structured interventions targeting life stories.

How should SLPs approach this challenge? A good starting point is learning more about why narrative is such an important part of the social fabric of our lives. We have much to learn from other disciplines. Each clinician can and should reflect on the role of story in her own life and the way that the small and big stories each of us tells provide opportunities to frame and validate our sense of who we are, our identity, as described further in Strong and Shadden (2020). Clinicians should also be more attentive to who they listen to, what they listen for, and how they listen when stories are being shared.

LPAA's influence on how we serve people living with aphasia has been profound. At the heart of this influence is the recognition that successful living with aphasia is grounded in social interaction, and that this social grounding serves complex functions. Our title captures our message that small and big stories are the currency we use to make meaning in our lives and to continually reframe our sense of who we are and where we are going. We hope the reader will respond to our call to action to be more attentive to story in the lives of our clients and their loved ones and to join in the honor of sharing our space with their stories.

References

Atkinson, R. (2002). The life story interview. In J. F. Gubrium & J. A. Holstein (Eds.), *Handbook of interview research: Content and method* (pp. 121–140). Thousand Oaks, CA: Sage.

Bamberg, M. (2012). Why narrative? *Narrative Inquiry, 22*(1), 202–210. https://doi.org/10.1075/ni.22.1.16bam

Beach, M. C., Inui, T., & the Relationship-Centered Care Network (2006). Relationship-centered care: A constructive reframing. *Journal of General Internal Medicine, 21*(S1), S3–S8. https://doi.org/10.1111/j.1525-1497.2006.00302.x

Birren, J. E., & Cochran, K. N. (2001). *Telling the stories of life through guided autobiography groups* (3rd ed.). Baltimore, MD: Johns Hopkins.

Bronken, B. A., Kirkevold, M., Martinsen, R., & Kvigne, K. (2012). The aphasic storyteller: Coconstructing stories to promote psychosocial well-being after stroke. *Qualitative Health Research, 22*(10), 1303–1316. https://doi.org/10.1177/1049732312450366

Buck, M. (1963). The language disorders: A personal and professional account of aphasia. *Journal of Rehabilitation, 29*, 37–38.

Bruner, J. (1999). Narratives of aging. *Journal of Aging Studies, 13*, 7–10. https://doi.org/10.1016/S0890-4065(99)80002-4

Charon, R., & Montello, M. (Eds.) (2002). *Stories matter: The role of narrative in medical ethics.* New York, NY: Routledge.

Corsten, S., Schimpf, E. J., Konradi, J., Keilmann, A., & Hardering, F. (2015). The participants' perspective: How biographic-narrative intervention influences identity negotiation and quality of life in aphasia. *International Journal of Language and Communication Disorders, 50*(6), 788–800. https://doi.org/10.1111/1460-6984.12173

Dipper, L., & Cruice, M. (2018). Personal storytelling in aphasia: A single case study of LUNA therapy. *Aphasiology, 32*(S1), 60–61. https://www.tandfonline.com/doi/full/10.1080/02687038.2018.1487919

Elman, R. J. (Ed.) (2007). *Group treatment of neurogenic communication disorders: The expert clinician's approach* (2nd ed.). San Diego, CA: Plural Publishing.

Ellis-Hill, C., Payne, S., & Ward, C. (2008). Using stroke to explore the life thread model: An alternative approach to understanding rehabilitation following acquired disability. *Disability and Rehabilitation, 30*(2), 150–159. https://doi.org/10.1080/09638280701195462

Frank, A. W. (2007). Just listening: Narrative and deep illness. In S. Krippner, M. Bova, & L. Gray (Eds.). Healing stories: The use of narrative in counseling and psychotherapy. (pp. 21–40). Charlottesville, VA: Puente Publications.

Frank, A. W. (2013). *The wounded storyteller.* Chicago, IL: University of Chicago Press.

Gubrium, J. F., & Holstein, J. A. (1998). Narrative practice and the coherence of personal stories. *The Sociological Quarterly, 39*(1), 163–187.

Hallé, M., LeDorze, G., & Mingant, A. (2014). Speech-language therapists' process of including significant others in aphasia rehabilitation. *International Journal of Language and Communication Disorders, 49*(6), 748–760. https://doi.org/10.1111/1460-6984.12108

Harari, Y. N. (2015). *Sapiens: A brief history of humankind.* New York, NY: HarperCollins.

Harris, J. L. (1997). Reminiscence: A culturally and developmentally appropriate language intervention for older adults. *American Journal of Speech-Language Pathology, 6*(3), 19–26. https://doi.org/10.1044/1058-0360.0603.19

Hersh, D. (2015). "Hopeless, sorry, hopeless": Co-constructing narratives of care with people who have aphasia post-stroke. *Topics in Language Disorders, 35*(3), 219–236. https://doi.org/10.1097/TLD.0000000000000060

Hinckley, J. (2007). *Narrative-based practice in speech-language pathology: Stories of a clinical life.* San Diego, CA: Plural Publishing.

Holland, A. L., & Nelson, R. L. (2018). *Counseling in communication disorders* (3rd ed.). San Diego, CA: Plural Publishing.

Holstein, J. A., & Gubrium, J. F. (2000). *The self we live by: Narrative identity in a postmodern world.* New York, NY: Oxford University Press.

Howe, T., Davidson, B., Worrall, L., Hersh, D., Ferguson, A., Sherratt, S., & Gilbert, J. (2012). "You needed to rehab . . . families as well": Family members' own goals for aphasia rehabilitation. *International Journal of Language and Communication Disorders, 47*(5), 511–521. https://doi.org/10.1111/j.1460-6984.2012.00159.x

Hyden, L. C. (1997). Illness and narrative. *Sociology of Health & Illness, 19*(1), 48–69. https://doi.org/10.1111/j.1467-9566.1997.tb00015

Hyden, L. C., (2008). Narratives in illness: A methodological note. *Qualitative Sociology Review, 5*(3), 49–58.

Keegan, C. (2013, Spring). Therapeutic writing: Life stories punctuated by healing. *Stroke Connection,* pp. 14–15.

Kenyon, G. M. (2003). Telling and listening to stories: Creating a wisdom environment for older people. *Generations, 27,* 30–43.

LeDorze, G. Tremblay, V., & Croteau, C. (2009). A qualitative longitudinal case of a daughter's adaptation process to her father's aphasia and stroke. *Aphasiology, 23,* 483–502. https://doi.org/10.1080/02687030801890909

LPAA Project Group (Chapey, R., Duchan, J., Elman, R., Garcia, L., Kagan, A., Lyon, J., & Simmons-Mackie, N.). (2000). Life participation approach to aphasia: A statement of values. *ASHA Leader, 5*(3), 4–6. https://doi.org/10.1044/leader.FTR.05032000.4

Lucius-Hoene, G., Holmberg, C., & Meyer, T. (2018). *Illness narratives in practice: Potentials and challenges of using narratives in health-related contexts.* Oxford, UK: Oxford University Press.

Lund, A., Melhus, M., & Sveen, U. (2017). Enjoyable company in sharing stroke experiences: Lifestyle groups after stroke. *Scandinavian Journal of Occupational Therapy, 25*(2), 127–135. https://doi.org/10.1080/11038128.2017.1341958

McAdams, D. P. (1997). *Guided autobiography. Northwestern University Foley Center for the Study of Lives*. Retrieved from https://www.sesp.northwestern.edu/foley/instruments/guided/

McAdams, D. P. (2008). Personal narratives and the life story. In O. John, R. W. Robins, & L. A. Pervin (Eds.). *Handbook of personality: Theory and research* (3rd ed., pp. 242–262). New York, NY: Guilford Press.

McAdams, D. P. (2018). Narrative identity: What is it? What does it do? How do you measure it? *Imagination, Cognition, and Personality: Consciousness in Theory, Research, and Clinical Practice, 37*(3), 339–372. https://doi.org/10.1177/0276236618756704

Natterlund, B. (2010). Being a close relative of a person with aphasia. *Scandinavian Journal of Occupational Therapy, 17*, 18–28. https://doi.org/10.3109/11038120902833218

Northcott, S., Moss, B., Harrison, K., & Hilari, K. (2015). A systematic review of the impact of stroke on social support and social networks: Associated factors and patterns of change. *Clinical Rehabilitation, 30*(8), 811–831. https://doi.org/10.1177/0269215515602136

Pluta, A., Ulatowska, H., Gawron, N., Sobanska, M., & Lojek, E. (2014). A thematic framework of illness narratives produced by stroke patients. *Disability and Rehabilitation, 37*(13), 1170–1177. https://www.tandfonline.com/doi/abs/10.3109/09638288.2014.957789

Randall, W. L., & Kenyon, G. M. (2000). *Ordinary wisdom: Biographical aging and the journey of life*. Westport, CT: Praeger.

Randall, W. L., Prior, S. M., & Skaborn, M. (2006). How listeners shape what tellers tell: Patterns of interaction in life story interviews and their impact on reminiscence by elderly interviewees. *Journal of Aging Studies, 20*(4), 381–396. https://doi.org/10.1016/j.jaging.2005.11.005

Rappaport, J. (1993). Narrative studies, personal stories, and identity transformation in the mutual help context. *Journal of Applied Behavioral Science, 29*, 239–256. https://doi.org/10.1177/0021886393292007

Richman, M. S., & Hartman, K. M. (2013, November). *Using guided autobiography in stroke survivor writing groups*. Seminar presented to the American Speech-Language-Hearing Association Convention, Chicago, IL.

Ryan, B., Worrall, L., Skehon, J., Baker, C. Carragher, M., Bohan, J., . . . Kneebone, I. (2020). Time to step up: A call for the speech pathology profession to utilise psychological care for people with aphasia post stroke. In K. H. Meredith & G. N. Yeates (Eds.), *Psychotherapy and aphasia* (pp. 1–16). New York, NY: Routledge.

Shadden, B. B. (2007). Rebuilding identity through stroke support groups: Embracing the person with aphasia and significant others. In R. Elman (Ed.), *Group treatment of neurogenic communication disorders: The expert clinician's approach* (2nd ed., pp.113–128). San Diego, CA: Plural Publishing.

Shadden, B. B., & Agan, J. P. (2004). Renegotiation of identity: The social context of aphasia support groups. *Topics in Language Disorders, 24*, 174–186.

Shadden, B. B., & Hagstrom, F. (2007). The role of narrative in the Life Participation Approach to Aphasia. *Topics in Language Disorders, 27*(4), 324–338. https://doi.org/10.1097/01.TLD.0000299887.24241.39

Shadden, B. B., Hagstrom, F., & Koski, P. R., (2008). *Neurogenic communication disorders: Life stories and the narrative self.* San Diego, CA: Plural Publishing.

Shadden, B. B., & Koski, P. (2007). Social construction of self for persons with aphasia: When language as a cultural tool is impaired. *Journal of Medical Speech-Language Pathology, 15*(2), 99–105.

Simmons-Mackie, N. (2018). *Aphasia in North America: Frequency, demographics, impact of aphasia, communication access services and service gaps.* Available at http://www.aphasiaaccess.org

Simmons-Mackie, N., & Elman, R. J. (2011). Negotiation of identity in group therapy: The Aphasia Café. *International Journal of Language & Communication Disorders, 46*(3), 321–323. https://doi.org/10.31 09/13682822.2010.507616

Strong, K. A. (2015). *Co-construction of personal narratives in supporting identity and communication in adults with aphasia: The 'My Story' Project* (Doctoral dissertation). Retrieved from Scholarworks https://scholarworks.wmich.edu/dissertations/748

Strong, K. A., Lagerwey, M. D., & Shadden, B. B. (2018). More than a story: My life came back to life. *American Journal of Speech-Language Pathology, 27*(IS), 464–476. https://doi.org/10.1044/2017_AJSLP-16-0167

Strong, K. A., & Nelson, N.W. (2012, November). *Supporting identity in aphasia: A survey of speech-language pathologists.* Poster presented to the American Speech-Language-Hearing Association Annual Convention, Atlanta, GA.

Strong, K. A., & Shadden, B. B. (2020). The power of story in identity renegotiation: Clinical approaches to supporting persons living with aphasia. *Perspectives of the ASHA Special Interest Groups.* https://doi.org/10.1044/2019_PERSP-19-00145

Taylor, C. (1994). The politics of recognition. In A. Gutman (Ed.) *Multiculturalism* (pp. 35–73). Princeton, NJ: Princeton University Press.

Ulatowska, J. K., Reyes, B., Santos, T. O., Garst, D., Vernon, J., & McArthur J. (2013). Personal narratives in aphasia: Understanding narrative competence. *Topics in Stroke Rehabilitation*, *20*(1), 36–43. https://doi.org/10.1310/tsr2001-36

Worrall, L., Davidson, B., Hersh, D., Howe, T., Sherratt, S., & Ferguson, A. (2010). The evidence for relationship-centered practice in aphasia rehabilitation. *Journal of Interactional Research in Communication Disorders*, *1*(2), 277–299. https://doi.org/10.1558/jircd.v1i2.277

World Health Organization. (2003). *The social determinants of health: The solid facts* (2nd ed.). Copenhagen, Denmark: WHO Regional Office for Europe. Available at http://www.euro.who.int/__data/assets/pdf_file/0005/98438/e81384.pdf

6

PRIMARY PROGRESSIVE APHASIA

A Practical Roadmap for Navigating Person-Centered Evaluation and Treatment

Rebecca Khayum and Aimee R. Mooney

Introduction

Our ability to communicate through spoken and written language is a quality that helps to define us as human beings. Imagine a disease that slowly strips away the ability to speak, read and write, while insight remains intact. Imagine receiving a diagnosis where you are told that someday, you may not be able to speak. Imagine being told that there is no cure for this illness. For people diagnosed with primary progressive aphasia (PPA), this difficult scenario becomes a reality. Many have traveled a long and complicated path to receive their diagnosis. Families living with PPA have often experienced significant emotional, financial, and occupational burden prior to even receiving the diagnosis. Resources and support may be difficult to find, particularly in rural areas.

With this devastating diagnosis comes an opportunity: An opportunity for speech-language pathologists (SLPs) to fill a current void in care. SLPs can provide the critical support that families living with PPA are seeking through aphasia-friendly disease education and counseling, communication strategy training, conversation partner training, and connection with local resources and programs. Perhaps most importantly, SLPs can offer reassurance that the diagnosis doesn't define them as a person. The Life Participation Approach to Aphasia (LPAA) offers a holistic, client-directed approach to treating people living with PPA. Using this intervention, SLPs foster communication confidence and resilience, and illustrate how meaningful moments can still occur during participation in desired activities and conversations with family and friends.

What Is Primary Progressive Aphasia?

Primary progressive aphasia (PPA) is a neurodegenerative dementia syndrome, characterized by a progressive decline in language abilities, with the preservation of other cognitive domains in the early stages. The syndrome was first described by Marsel Mesulam (1982). This aphasic dementia may impact expressive language, receptive language, reading, and writing abilities (Mesulam, Wieneke, Thompson, Rogalski, & Weintraub, 2012). Although PPA can be diagnosed at any age, it is considered an early onset dementia, with the onset of symptoms most frequently occurring between the ages of 50 and 70 years (Croot, 2009; Mesulam, Rogalski & Wieneke, 2014). PPA is a clinical diagnosis, meaning that it describes the initial symptoms the person is experiencing. PPA is considered a form of frontotemporal dementia because the initial atrophy typically occurs in the left frontotemporal region of the brain. All dementia syndromes get worse over time, as atrophy spreads. Therefore, although language is initially affected in PPA, other nonlanguage cognitive areas will be impacted over time (Mesulam, Rogalski, & Wieneke, 2014).

One may be asking, what is causing the brain atrophy? This leads to the second diagnosis a person living with PPA may receive: the suspected neuropathological diagnosis. In simple terms, misfolded proteins that aggregate over time lead to the neurodegeneration in the brain. The most common neuropathologic causes of PPA are frontotemporal lobar degeneration and Alzheimer's disease (Mesulam, Rogalski, & Wieneke, 2014). Of note, "Alzheimer's disease" refers to the neuropathologic diagnosis, while "Alzheimer's dementia" refers to the clinical diagnosis. Currently, the only way to accurately confirm the neuropathologic diagnosis is at autopsy; however, biomarkers are being developed, via amyloid or tau positron emission tomography (PET) and cerebrospinal fluid (Mesulam, Rogalski & Wieneke, 2014). A biomarker refers to something that can be accurately measured to indicate the presence of a disease. Why is knowing the neuropathology important? When disease-modifying drugs are eventually discovered, they will target the underlying pathology, not the clinical symptoms.

People living with PPA will often be labeled with a PPA subtype, particularly if diagnosed in the early stages. The three described subtypes or variants are semantic (PPA-S), agrammatic (PPA-G) *(also termed non-fluent variant)*, and logopenic (PPA-L; Gorno-Tempini et al., 2011). The semantic subtype is characterized by an impairment in the understanding of word meanings. Language is often fluent, but may increasingly lack content. The agrammatic subtype is characterized by symptoms of agrammatism in written and spoken language. Effortful or apraxic speech may also be present. The logopenic subtype is characterized by difficulties in lexical retrieval and deficits in repetition ability. Of note, for individuals who display symptoms of a progressive apraxia of speech in the absence of aphasia, the diagnosis of primary progressive apraxia of speech (PPAOS) may be appropriate (Duffy et al., 2015). Although PPA subtypes may be helpful in a research context, many people do not "fit neatly" into a subtype bin (Harris et al., 2013; Mesulam, Rogalski, et al., 2014). For example, a person may exhibit initial symptoms that meet the criteria for both PPA-L and PPA-G. In addition, symptoms change as the disease progresses, and people may often exhibit symptoms from multiple subtypes. Further, PPA subtype is not an accurate predictor of neuropathologic diagnosis, as there is no 1:1 correlation between subtype and neuropathology (Gorno-Tempini et al., 2011; Mesulam, Weintraub, et al., 2014).

People living with PPA and their family members may become confused and frustrated when they are diagnosed with one subtype by one professional and a different subtype by another professional. They may be told to expect particular symptoms to arise in the future, based upon their initial symptoms. However, more research is needed to understand the progression of symptoms; there is significant individual variability in rate of progression and emergence of new symptoms. SLPs should use caution in utilizing the subtype to guide disease education and counseling. Providing people living with PPA and their family members with inaccurate descriptions of what symptoms will "likely" occur down the road may cause unnecessary anxiety and fear. Although it is important for SLPs to be familiar with the different subtypes and to provide education and training to family members, it may be more helpful to look at symptom profiles over time, and how a person's unique symptoms are impacting functional communication in daily life situations. This chapter will provide practical suggestions to help SLPs to be mindful of PPA subtype while maintaining focus on LPAA assessment, goal formation, and intervention.

Readers may be wondering at this point, "Why all of this background information about PPA in a book about LPAA?" Why do SLPs need to know all of this information? Many people living with PPA and their families have received the diagnosis, but are lacking disease education, counseling, and support (Riedl, Last, Danek, & Diehl-Schmid, 2014). The SLP may be the first person who has the ability to explain their diagnosis in an aphasia-friendly way, while empathizing with the burden and loss that they are experiencing. SLPs must have a thorough understanding of PPA in order to be truly effective in helping those diagnosed to meet their communication participation goals.

Counseling and Support: It Takes a Team

Many health care professionals aren't familiar with PPA, so it is ideal if SLPs can help refer families to a local neurologist or specialists at Alzheimer's disease Centers to receive a thorough neurological work up and accurate diagnosis. Readers can find a list of federally funded Alzheimer's Disease Centers at https://www.nia.nih.gov/health/alzheimers-disease-research-centers

There are many professionals who may be a part of the person's care team: behavioral neurologists, neuropsychologists, psychologists, psychiatrists, social workers, physical therapists, and occupational therapists. Using an interdisciplinary approach to care, with the person's and family's concerns and needs driving the treatment, is important to help manage the complex needs of individuals with this younger onset dementia syndrome (Morhardt et al., 2015). With the average survival of 7 to 10 years, and a documented range of 2 to 20 years, ongoing support and resources will be required to meet a person's changing needs (Dickerson, 2011; Diehl-Schmid et al., 2007).

It is important to understand how the person living with PPA and family members are coping with the diagnosis. Asking questions such as, "Tell me about your understanding of PPA," and then, "How much would you like to know?" gives SLPs an opportunity to listen, empathize, and counsel. People living with PPA experience a higher rate of depression than those living with Alzheimer's dementia due to their preserved insight (Medina & Weintraub, 2007). Referral to social workers, psychologists, and psychiatrists to manage symptoms of depression and anxiety may be a critical step in preparation for effective participation in speech-language therapy sessions. In addition to providing psychosocial support, social workers may provide resources to help families prepare for the future (Morhardt, O'Hara, Zachrich, Wieneke, & Rogalski, 2017). Elder law attorneys, financial advisors, adult day programs, caregiver companies, home health agencies, and hospice agencies may all offer support to help families navigate the difficult road ahead.

Assessment: Diagnostic or Person-Centered Treatment Planning

For SLPs working on diagnostic teams, utilizing a battery of impairment-based standardized tests may be helpful in making an accurate diagnosis. Henry and Grasso provide a comprehensive review of diagnostic assessment in PPA (Henry & Grasso, 2018). For SLPs tasked with the goal of developing person-centered, functional plans of care, the use of these same standardized tests will result in a purpose-product mismatch. Alternative approaches that "flip the rehab model" and focus on client-directed care may be helpful frameworks for conducting an LPAA-focused evaluation for people living with a progressive aphasia (Bourgeois, 2014). Traditional rehabilitation approaches focus upon identifying the person's impairments through standardized testing and then implementing clinician-directed interventions to target the impaired domains. Bourgeois suggests that SLPs should flip this model for a client-directed approach: assessment should start with motivational interviewing of the person living with dementia, along with family and staff members, to determine how the impairments are impacting participation in daily conversations and life activities. As Kagan and Simmons-Mackie and colleagues suggest, SLPs should consider "beginning at the end" when it comes to LPAA assessment (2008).

By starting with a thorough interview of the person living with PPA and their communication partner, SLPs create an intervention plan driven by functional participation goals. One tool to administer to accomplish this goal is the The Social Networks Inventory (SNI) (Blackstone & Hunt-Berg, 2003). The SNI was developed to provide a framework to understand each person's circle of communication partners, the types and variety of communication modalities used with each partner, and common topics chosen during conversation. The goal is to help individuals, practitioners and family members develop a current picture of an individual's daily communication life, including opportunities and barriers to participation in the life activities resulting from PPA. The SNI is adaptable and does not need to be administered in its entirety. Results will inform what modes of communication are being used, how they can be expanded or optimized to different partners or environments, and communication partner training needs. Fried-Oken reassures that SLPs are then equipped with the understanding where and when communication challenges exist so that they can find ways to place the person's "mental dictionary" in front of them, allowing them to participate in daily activities as his/her language skills decline (Fried-Oken, 2008).

Client-Reported Outcome Measures and Goal Writing

Insurance reimbursement relies upon the SLP's ability to demonstrate progress, often through the use of standardized test scores. For people living with a neurodegenerative disease, obtaining the same score pre- and posttreatment may actually indicate progress, because one would expect the score to decline over time. This dilemma begs the question: how do SLPs demonstrate progress for people living with PPA, to ensure insurance reimbursement for treatment? Standardized tests that focus upon context-based communication tasks, such as the Communication Activities of Daily Living (CADL-3; Holland, Fromm & Wozniak, 2018), or the Assessment of Language-Related Functional Activities (ALFA; Baines, Martin, & Heeringa, 1999), may certainly be helpful. In addition, integrating measures that capture the client's self-reported outcomes may help to demonstrate progress toward LPAA goals. Examples are the Assessment for Living with Aphasia (ALA; Simmons-Mackie et al., 2014) or the Communication Confidence Rating Scale for Aphasia (CCRSA; Babbit, Heinemann, Semik, & Cherney, 2011).

SLP intervention goals need to be based on current assessment information, and relevant to people living with PPA and their communication partners. When carefully chosen and written in the SMARTER goal setting framework, (Shared, Monitored, Accessible, Relevant, Transparent, Evolving, and Relationship-centered) the person living with PPA can make progress toward carefully selected goals. Remembering that both direct and indirect interventions are validated by the American Speech-Language-Hearing Association (ASHA), goals may target strategies that are being implemented by the communication partner to facilitate communication (Hopper et al., 2013). Frequency counts of the behaviors of interest, the amount of assistance or cues required to perform a task, the number and type of errors made during an activity, and the nature of the partner's communication behaviors are all appropriate outcome measures. Given the degenerative nature of PPA, global measures of communication or cognitive function will not be sensitive to improvements in specific skills or behaviors that occur as a result of interventions.

Language Interventions for People Living with PPA

Research evidence to support language intervention in PPA is emerging; evidence remains limited in comparison to literature in stroke-induced aphasia. An increasing number of recent studies investigating impairment-based interventions for word retrieval are revealing promising results on treated word items but with limited impact on generalization. Systematic reviews of word retrieval interventions (semantic and phonological treatments) indicate immediate gains, but the question remains as to whether people living with PPA maintain these gains over time and if the gains generalize to functional contexts (Cadorio, Lousada, Martins, & Figueiredo, 2017; Croot, Nickels, Laurence, & Manning, 2009; Jokel, Graham, Rochon, & Leonard, 2014). Several studies have incorporated personally relevant stimuli into session and home practice, to promote generalization and maintenance in daily conversations (Henry et al., 2019; Rogalski et al., 2016). Other studies have examined the effects of oral reading treatment and script practice on speech production and fluency. Positive gains were documented on the trained content following treatment (Henry et al., 2013a; Henry et al., 2018).

Volkmer and colleagues completed a systematic review of 19 studies targeting functional communication interventions for people living with PPA and their care partners (2019). Although there was much variation in location, dosage, and intensity of treatment, analysis indicated two common components of functional interventions: (1) reinforcing and strengthening communication skills that the person living with PPA is already comfortable using; and (2) incorporating communication partner (CP) training throughout treatment to encourage generalization of communication strategies.

Evidence is building for participation-level interventions that focus on development and utilization of Augmentative and Alternative Communication (AAC) strategies to maximize communication (Khayum et al., 2012; Mooney, Bedrick, Noethe, Spaulding, & Fried-Oken, 2018; Mooney, Beale, & Fried-Oken, 2018). Success has been reported in training communication boards/books or other low-tech AAC in anticipation of potential language decline (Kortte & Rogalski, 2013).

Effective communication treatment in degenerative language loss is based on two principles: (1) treatment must be provided early and over the course of disease progression (Croot et al., 2009; Fried-Oken, Beukelman, & Hux, 2012; Jokel et al., 2014; Rogers, King, & Alarcon, 2000) and (2) communication partners are key components of intervention at every stage (Beukelman, Garrett, & Yorkston, 2007; Pattee, Von Berg, & Ghezzi, 2006; Rogers & Alarcon, 1998). Communication partners play an essential role in the lives of people living with PPA. As a person loses skills, the partner assumes more responsibility for communicative interaction and message coconstruction (Fried-Oken, 2008). As often as feasible, SLPs must include communication partners in treatment sessions. After determining functional participation goals, AAC strategies can be identified and systematically trained. Through repeated practice, this person-centered intervention provides the dyad with real hope of maintaining social interactions in a variety of environments, even in the face of disease progression.

Group therapy models have also been studied in people living with PPA, targeting a range of topics including: disease education, support and counseling, communication strategy training, and social activities (language or non-language based). Studies found that people living with PPA and their family members demonstrated increased confidence and felt valued after group participation (Jokel & Meltzer, 2017; Kim, Figeys, Hubbard, & Wilson, 2018; Mooney, Beale, & Fried-Oken, 2018; Morhardt et al.,

2017). Additional positive outcomes included improvements in quality of communication and coping skills when compared to matched controls who did not receive group intervention.

There is a paucity of LPAA-guided models for PPA intervention in the literature. The Communication Bridge Care Model introduced a person-centered care model which focused on dyadic instruction for disease education, paired with a unique combination of personalized impairment-based exercises and compensatory strategy training for 34 dyads living with PPA. Goals were client-directed and aimed to increase participation (Rogalski et al., 2016; Rogalski & Khayum, 2018). This person-centered model indicated that it is feasible to provide LPAA-focused speech-language treatment via telehealth and that participants demonstrated increased confidence in their communication skills.

In summary, more research is needed to investigate the efficacy of various language interventions for people living with PPA. The remainder of this chapter will consider how to apply the current evidence to support LPAA-focused care.

Blending a Variety of Interventions to Support LPAA Goals

An LPAA-driven care model may incorporate many interventions to support client-directed, participation goals. A combination of disease education, counseling, personalized impairment-based exercises, compensatory strategies, and environmental modifications may all be utilized to support a client's goals.

Disease Education and Counseling

For disease education and counseling, SLPs should ensure that the person living with PPA and family members understand the diagnosis, while linking the person and family members with other health care professionals and local resources for ongoing support. The SLP may also introduce options of how to share the PPA diagnosis or education about aphasia with family, friends, and strangers. For example, the SLP may provide a card that explains the condition for use with others, script practice to relay important information about PPA, and develop letters and e-mails designed for family members and friends. Here are some helpful counseling tips when working with people living with PPA and their family members:

- Always be on the lookout for potential "counseling moments." These moments will require the SLP to pause, listen, empathize, and validate as needed (Holland & Nelson, 2018).
- Don't be afraid to say, "I don't know." People living with PPA and their family members may have questions such as: How quickly will this progress? What symptoms will develop next? Will I not be able to speak at all someday? Will my swallowing become effected? Will his personality change over time? Will she have difficult behaviors like people with Alzheimer's dementia? Unfortunately, there is no way to accurately answer these questions. It's important to acknowledge the question and the pain behind it. SLPs can also reassure that these questions are the current focus of much research, and we hope to have answers in the future. In the meantime, the best way for families living with PPA to optimize participation is to prepare for potential changes in language function by learning strategies that will address any symptoms that do arise over time. We hope they may not need all of the strategies, but it is the SLP's job to ensure they are prepared.
- It is ok to pause an SLP session to provide support when the person living with PPA or their communication partner becomes tearful.
    - Let them know that they aren't in this journey alone.
    - Recognize the enormous burden placed on the person and their family through use of validation statements such as, "I can see how difficult/frustrating this must be for you," "I want to thank you for sharing this with me," "I understand what you're saying," or "I am so sorry you are going through this . . . know that I am here with you."
- Be comfortable with silence.

- Recognize that you can't "fix" PPA; rather, SLPs are partners in helping to manage symptoms as they present themselves.
  - SLPs are problem solvers. When working with people who have stroke-induced aphasia, there is always the goal of "getting better" and improving skills over time. Counseling for people living with PPA will differ in that their symptoms will not get better over time. It is important to acknowledge the gravity of your client's situation, empathize with them, and not immediately jump to strategies that will "fix" the communication difficulties.

Impairment-Based Interventions

Personalized impairment-based exercises may be targeted to help restore lexical retrieval, fluency/motor speech production, reading and writing for daily conversations and functional tasks. Examples of restorative interventions include: lexical retrieval cascade treatment (Henry et al., 2013b), generative naming tasks, motor speech strategies (e.g., oral reading treatment with syllable segmentation (Henry et al., 2013a), fading cues hierarchy for apraxia of speech (Rosenbek et al., 1973), melodic and rhythmic strategies (Beber et al., 2018), script practice (with video articulatory cues if needed; Youmans, Holland, Munoz, & Bourgeois, 2005), Copy and Recall Treatment for writing (CART; Beeson & Egnor, 2006) or Oral Reading for Language in Aphasia (ORLA; Cherney, 2010).

Compensatory Interventions

Compensatory approaches provide people living with PPA and their family members with a toolbox of strategies to enhance functional communication. Compensatory approaches may include conversation training with communication partners, such as the Supported Conversation for Adults with Aphasia (SCA™) program, which trains the person living with PPA and their communication partner to use strategies such as keywords, body language and gestures, hand drawing, and visual aids to "keep the conversation alive" (Kagan, 1998). SLPs may introduce the use of low-tech and high-tech alternative-augmentative communication (AAC) to supplement verbal language. AAC may include native/built-in apps (apps that come preloaded on mobile technology) on smart phone or tablet, communication apps on smart phone or tablet, a communication book or wallet, key word visual aids, or a speech generating device (SGD).

Environmental Modifications

Training in environmental modifications to enhance communication may also be helpful. The environment may be modified to optimize comprehension of daily conversations by training the person living with PPA and their communication partner to eliminate distractions, sit in a quiet corner in restaurants, and to communicate face to face while making eye contact. The strategic placement of visual communication aids around the environment can help to facilitate optimal use during conversations.

Personalized Lexicons

SLPs can help people living with PPA and their family members create a "mini-lexicon" of salient words and phrases used in daily conversations (Fried-Oken, 2008). This process may take place over several sessions, as SLPs facilitate the brainstorming process. Completing generative naming tasks for different semantic categories can help to strategically generate the mini-lexicon. The categories may include: people (family members, friends, neighbors, coworkers, doctors); places (stores, restaurants, street names, important countries, states, cities); food and beverages; household objects and devices; hobbies/interests (sports, movies, books, current events, politics, travel, etc.); and long-term care setting vocabulary (staff member and resident names, common requests, building activities and locations). The mini-lexicon can be stored and used to create personally relevant word rehearsal programs and the content for scripts and communication visual supports (communication books, wallets, or words in communication app/speech generating device).

A variety of interventions may be applied to meet participation goals in Table 6–1.

Table 6–1. Participation Goals

Participation Goal	Impairment Interventions	Compensatory Interventions
Engaging in conversations with CP or healthcare staff	• Salient word/phrase rehearsal program targeting daily conversation topics • Script rehearsal	• Conversation training with CP/staff members • Key word visual aids • "Main topic" visual aid • Script visual aids • Communication book/wallet • Training use of photo stream and native apps to support conversation • Create visual sequencing aids for activities of daily living (ADLs)
Engaging in group conversations at weekly book club, lunch group, or group activity in assisted living setting	• Salient word/phrase rehearsal relevant topics • Script rehearsal for discussion responses	• Educate group members about PPA • Conversation training with leader and members of group • Environmental modifications: selecting quiet restaurant, seating arrangement • Look up online menu in advance: write out order and use visual aid to place order • Plan ahead: write out and rehearse discussion points • Key wording: make visual aid with key words for lunch conversation or for characters/plot points • Use of AAC as needed—photo stream, key words in "notes" app, remnants

Participation Goal	Impairment Interventions	Compensatory Interventions
Talking on the phone with family and friends; taking phone messages	• Salient word/phrase rehearsal for words related to family/friends and activities • Script rehearsal	• Consider using video chat instead of audio call (e.g., FaceTime® or Skype®) • Conversation Training with family/friends • Use of visual communication supports during call—key word visual aid, script aid • Visual script aid next to phone that states: "I don't have a pen handy … could you please call back and leave a voicemail with the information?" or "Please repeat that again slowly. I need to write it down." • Phone message template, listing frequent callers (family, friends, doctors) and common reasons they are calling.
Increasing independence in meal planning and preparation	• Salient word/phrase and script rehearsal for common food items	• Create weekly meal planning visual aid, to plan recipes for each day • Create aphasia-friendly recipes: select client's favorite recipes and re-write each step into short phrase, with accompanying pictures • Create grocery list visual aid of typical groceries/items purchased each week • Create visual aids and organizational systems for food organization in pantry and fridge

continues

145

Table 6–1. *continued*

Participation Goal	Impairment Interventions	Compensatory Interventions
Writing emails, text messages, or Facebook posts or greeting cards more quickly and with greater accuracy	• CART—written practice of common words/phrases used for texts, emails, cards	• Use of voice recognition technology (VRT) to dictate verbal message into text • Training consistent use of spell/grammar check and word prediction • Using app such as Grammarly® to correct spelling and grammar • CP training—working as a team to compose text messages/emails and proofreading • Increasing use of pictures/emoji's to help communicate message • For greeting cards, use visual templates to copy people's names, common messages. • Signature stamp
Reading novels, magazines, or newspaper articles for pleasure	• Paragraph re-reading for comprehension (SQ3R method)	• Read paperback book while listening to audio book version to aid comprehension • Modify reading content: select familiar authors or novels; novels containing short stories; magazines with large print and numerous pictures (e.g., Reader's Digest® or National Geographic®) • Try aphasia-friendly news source, such as Lingraphica's Newspath®. • For e-books: highlight difficult words to pull up picture and definition for single word comprehension • Write key words/characters on index cards to aid comprehension

Staying One Step Ahead

After reviewing the chart listing LPAA goals and interventions, many SLPs may be asking, "How do these goals and interventions differ from people with stroke-induced aphasia?" Indeed, the same chart may be applicable for targeting life participation goals in the stroke-induced aphasia population; however, the application of the interventions over time is drastically different for people living with PPA. Although more research is needed to determine appropriate intensity and frequency of speech-language intervention for those living with PPA, there are two important considerations when working this population. The first is the difference in symptom onset. People living with stroke-induced aphasia have typically experienced an abrupt loss of language abilities, whereas people living with PPA have been gradually coping with a decline in their language skills. By the time a person living with PPA meets with an SLP, he or she has likely developed many compensatory strategies over the past several years to help with speaking, comprehension, writing, and reading. SLPs should take a full inventory of communication strategies that are already in use, encourage the continued use of effective strategies, and build upon this strategy toolbox to meet a person's changing needs over time.

The second difference from working with the stroke-induced aphasia population is the importance of modifying communication strategies over time, as a person's speaking, comprehension, reading, and/or writing skills decline. A person may have the same life participation goal (e.g., having a back and forth conversation with a spouse or participating in a book club), but a unique combination of strategies and level of communication partner (CP) support will be required to meet this goal. SLPs should carefully consider a person's communication strengths versus challenges, and utilize the preserved strengths to help with compensation. It is also critical to anticipate language decline, and introduce new communication tools before they are actually needed. For example, preemptively introducing the use of high- or low-tech AAC supports may help to promote more effective use over time. Getting buy-in for compensatory strategies will be different for everyone. Building upon the person's strengths when introducing new tools may be helpful. For example, if a client enjoys taking photos on her smart phone, the SLP could train the strategic use of the photos during daily conversations. If a client is reluctant to use a picture-based support, perhaps he would be willing to refer to a written list of important people and places to help with retrieval during conversations.

The SLP's role is to establish a relationship with people with PPA and their families, similar to a dental care model: "We are in this together; I'd like to plan on seeing you every 6 months (or in some cases, less), just as you would see a dentist for preventative or maintenance care." SLPs may have a short, intensive period of intervention to train a new compensatory strategy or provide conversation partner training. Once the new skills are mastered, treatment intensity could decrease for the subsequent sessions targeting maintenance and generalization. Once generalization is achieved, the SLP can advise the person living with PPA and their communication partner to consider scheduling an evaluation whenever changes in communication are noted in the future.

Are the Communication Strategies Generalizing?

An important question for a population who experiences a progressive decline in language skills is: *"How can I ensure that communication strategies are generalized and maintained over time?"* The first consideration should be the instructional approach. Too often SLPs limit visits with individuals with degenerative disease thinking they have made suggestions, given strategy recommendations and have nothing left to offer. It is vital that these suggestions and strategies are trained to mastery and then to generalization. Solberg and Turkstra (2011) give excellent models of systematic instruction principles to ensure treatment is effective for clients with cognitive-communication disorders. Assistive technology without training is NOT assistive.

Another element to consider is the importance of ongoing CP involvement in treatment, while utilizing direct instruction for communication strategy training (Ehlhardt & Kennedy, 2005; Glang et al., 2008). Involving CPs in the initial speech-language assessment and throughout the plan of care ensures that a team approach is utilized when constructing client-directed, life participation goals and developing communication tools to target these goals. Because communication typically involves more than one person (unless you carry on most of your daily conversations with yourself), it is natural that CP involvement should be considered an integral component of treatment sessions, so ongoing education and training can be provided. As the client's language skills decline over time, increased support will be required from the CP to ensure effective communication.

Coordinating CP participation may be difficult with the PPA population because many experience the onset of symptoms at a younger age than Alzheimer's dementia. Spouses may still be working or children may not live locally, making it necessary for SLPs to think outside the box to involve CPs in treatment sessions. For example, perhaps the CP could join the session via an audio conference call or via video conferencing on days they cannot physically be present in the session. On days when a family member is unable to be present, SLPs could work with the person living with PPA to compose an email or record a short video on their phone, summarizing the session and what strategies to practice in the home environment. It is important to note that some people living with PPA may not have a close family member or support team involved in their care. In these situations, SLPs should coordinate with social workers and other health care providers to ensure the person is linked with resources that will provide the necessary support.

For people living in assisted living or long-term care, staff members (nursing staff, activities staff, caregivers) should be involved in education and training on supportive communication tools. SLPs can consider making a "communication station" in the person's room, where all communication aids are organized for easy access. Pulling staff members into five minutes of the therapy session for training on use of communication supports will help with generalization of the strategies. In applying the life participation approach in long term care, SLPs can also ensure that some treatment sessions take place during facility activities and events, to observe the person's functional communication in these environments. Communication tools can be personalized and adapted to meet their needs for specific activities. For example, SLPs can help to create visual communication aids for cooking club, book club, current events, choir, or exercise groups. The task of creating multiple aids may be daunting for busy SLPs; it is important to engage and train other family members and friends to help in this process and ensure generalization and maintenance.

Practical Tips for Creating Personalized Communication Supports During Therapy Sessions or Aphasia Groups

Technological advancement is enabling SLPs to develop personalized communication aids to support LPAA goals more easily. Whether working in an aphasia center, academic institution, support group, outpatient clinic, or in long-term care, SLPs must consider how development of personalized communication supports may help their client living with PPA meet their participation goals. Paper-based supports can be made as a team with the person living with PPA and family members. Communication wallets can be created using a slide creation program, such as Microsoft PowerPoint®. Slides can be printed two to four per page and then laminated, cut, and placed on a key ring. For personalized picture-based supports, a collage making program such as the Pic Collage® app may be helpful. SLPs can involve the person living with PPA in the formulation of the supports by selecting desired photos, determining best way to organize (sematic category or activity based), and assessing font size and contrast.

Thoughts on Use of Apps

Many people living with PPA and their family members may seek advice on "the best aphasia apps" to download. SLPs can provide education on how to strategically consider a unique variety of apps to meet participation goals. A combination of native/built-in apps, downloaded/purchased apps, and apps designed for communication/aphasia may provide the most support for individualized needs. Holland and colleagues discuss the importance of routinely searching for current or newly released apps that may be helpful in supporting a specific skill or participation goal (Holland, Weinberg, & Dittelman, 2012). For example, if the LPAA goal is hosting a holiday cookie exchange, the following apps could be utilized:

- Built-in app: "Notes" section of phone: Use key wording strategy to formulate lists of cookie recipes, ingredients, cooking utensils, and names of attendees. Print out and place in plastic page protector if needed.
- Built-in app: Photo stream: take screenshots of each type of cookie and the recipe for easy reference.
- Built-in app: Voice Recognition Technology (Siri®, Cortana®): Dictate words for e-mails and texts that are communicating information about the cookie exchange (to compensate for spelling difficulties).
- Downloaded app: Grammarly®: Assistance with correcting grammar and spelling errors for e-mails and texts that are communicating information about the cookie exchange.
- Downloaded app: Pinterest®: make a cookie recipe board.
- Downloaded app: Pic Collage®: make visual sequencing aids for cookie recipes, print out and place in page protector.

Think Twice Before Recommending that Device

Many people living with PPA and their family members may seek advice from an SLP on whether to consider a speech-generating device (SGD), knowing that verbal communication will become increasingly difficult down the road. Many factors should be considered before recommending the purchase of a high-tech SGD: (1) Client interest and motivation in using a high-tech device to communicate; (2) Client's prior experience with high tech devices; (3) Client's current ability to operate simple devices, such as a TV remote or microwave; (4) Communication partner support and familiarity with technology; (5) Presence of visual or fine motor deficits; (6) Impaired auditory comprehension or decreased ability to follow directions; (7) Presence of nonlanguage cognitive deficits (attention, sequencing, initiation) (Khayum et al., 2012).

Thoughtful considerations must be made as to whether the client is likely to use a SGD to communicate in the later stages, when other cognitive domains are also impaired. Working with the person living with PPA and family members to try out several devices before making a decision can help determine which device is a good fit. For people who are good candidates for a SGD, ordering the device before it is actually needed for communication may be helpful. This gives the person and family members time to program the device with personalized pictures and relevant phrases, while practicing use of the device during daily conversations. Some people may also be interested in "voice banking," which is the recording of personally relevant stories, phrases, and words in the earlier stages of PPA, in order to preserve the digital audio file for use as language declines.

Staying Integrated in the Community

In stroke-induced aphasia, LPAA interventions might aim to help an individual re-integrate into the community and social gatherings. For people living with PPA, the reverse situation is taking place: how can SLPs help their clients *stay* integrated in the community, as symptoms progress? Working collaboratively with the person living with PPA, their family members, and other health care professionals, SLPs can identify particular communication partners or settings where communication is becoming increasingly difficult and help to prevent social withdrawal by increasing communication confidence through the use of multicomponent, tailored interventions. Collaborating with social work to identify meaningful volunteer activities that take advantage of the person's preserved strengths may also help to prevent community withdrawal. For people living in long-term care, SLPs can work with the person, along with family and staff members, to identify meaningful roles and activities to participate in each day.

SLPs can also play a critical role in linking people living with PPA with local support groups, aphasia groups, or aphasia centers. Careful consideration should be given as to whether the local supports are a good fit. For example, will a person living with PPA and family members find benefit when participating in a dementia support group where most members are experiencing amnestic rather than language difficulties? Will they feel comfortable participating in an aphasia group where most members are living with stroke-induced aphasia and experience improvement rather than decline over time? Long-term participation of the PPA population in aphasia groups or centers also presents a dilemma to program facilitators if the person begins to exhibit behavioral or attentional symptoms that make it difficult for participation in program activities. More research is needed to investigate the potential advantages versus disadvantages of people living with PPA participating in predominantly stroke-induced aphasia programs. In the meantime, SLPs may want to consider an individualized approach when considering these different opportunities and openly discuss the pros and cons with family members. Having a person living with PPA participate in the program on a "trial basis" to determine if it's a good fit and then reassessing every six months may also help to overcome challenges. If a person no longer is appropriate for a particular aphasia group or center, the program coordinator can help link the family with another local program that would be better designed to fit their changing needs. It is also important to remind people living with PPA and their family members that there is significant individual variability in disease symptoms and progression, so that they are not attempting to compare themselves to other group members living with PPA.

Resilience

We have collectively worked with several hundred people living with PPA over the past 10 years. One common theme has presented itself: in the face of a devastating diagnosis, these individuals and families have revealed incredible resolve and resilience.

They have taught us much about life and overcoming seemingly insurmountable challenges. They have demonstrated how to live in the moment, while treasuring moments of joy and laugher, and how to find humor in the challenges. They have taught us to be grateful for the little things in life. They have taught us that it is ok to cry and admit that things are not ok. They have shown us the importance of asking for help and leaning on others in times of need. They have demonstrated compassion and selflessness when participating in PPA research: "I am participating in research and brain donation not because it will benefit me, but because I want to help others in the future." Although PPA may significantly impact the communication ability of these individuals, it cannot take away their incredible resilience. We are grateful for all that they have taught us and will continue to teach us until a cure is found.

References

Babbitt, E. M., Heinemann, A. W., Semik, P., & Cherney, L. R. (2011). Psychometric properties of the Communication Confidence Rating Scale for Aphasia (CCRSA): Phase 2. *Aphasiology, 25,* 727–735

Baines, K. A., Martin, A. W., & Heeringa, H. M. (1999). *LFA: The Assessment of Language-Related Functional Activities.* Austin, TX: Pro-Ed.

Beber, B. C., Berbert, M. C. B., Grawer, R. S., & Cardoso, M. C. A. F. (2018). Rate and rhythm control strategies for apraxia of speech in nonfluent primary progressive aphasia. *Dementia & Neuropsychologia, 12*(1), 80–84. https://doi.org/10.1590/1980-57642018dn12-010012

Beeson, P. M., & Egnor, H. (2006). Combining treatment for written and spoken naming. *Journal of the International Neuropsychological Society, 12*(6), 816–827.

Beukelman, D. R., Garrett, K. L., & Yorkston, K. M. (2007). *Augmentative communication strategies for adults with acute or chronic medical conditions.* Baltimore, MD: Brookes.

Blackstone, S. W., & Hunt-Berg, M. (2003). *Social Networks Inventory: A communication inventory for individuals with complex communication needs and their communication partners.* Verona, WI: Attainment Company.

Bourgeois, M. A. (2014, March). *Functional approach to assessment in dementia: Some new ideas.* Paper presented at ASHA Healthcare Conference, Las Vegas, NV.

Cadorio, I., Lousada, M., Martins, P., & Figueiredo, D. (2017). Generalization and maintenance of treatment gains in primary progressive aphasia (PPA): A systematic review. *International Journal of Language and Communication Disorders*, *52*(5), 543–560.

Cherney, L. R. (2010). Oral Reading for Language in Aphasia (ORLA): Evaluating the efficacy of computer-delivered therapy in chronic nonfluent aphasia. *Topics in Stroke Rehabilitation*, *17*(6), 423–431.

Croot, K. (2009). Progressive language impairments: Definitions, diagnoses, and prognoses. *Aphasiology*, *23*(2), 302–326.

Croot, K., Nickels, L., Laurence, F., & Manning, M. (2009). Impairment- and activity/participation-directed interventions in progressive language impairment: Clinical and theoretical issues. *Aphasiology*, *23*(2), 125–160.

Dickerson, B. C. (2011). Quantitating severity and progression in primary progressive aphasia. *Journal of Molecular Neuroscience*, *45*(3), 618–628.

Diehl-Schmid, J., Pohl, C., Perneczky, R., Hartmann, J., Forstl, H., & Kurz, A. (2007). Initial symptoms, survival and causes of death in 115 patient with frontotemporal lobar degeneration. *Fortschritte der Neurologie-Psychatrie*, *75*(12), 708–713.

Duffy, J. R., Strand, E. A., Clark, H., Machulda, M., Whitwell, J. L., & Josephs, K. A. (2015). Primary progressive apraxia of speech: Clinical features and acoustic and neurologic correlates, *American Journal of Speech-Language Pathology*, *24*(2), 88–100.

Ehlhardt, L., & Kennedy, M. (2005, November). Instructional techniques in cognitive rehabilitation: A preliminary report. *Seminars in Speech and Language*, *26*(4), 268–279.

Fried-Oken, M. (2008). Augmentative and alternative communication treatment for persons with primary progressive aphasia. *Perspectives on Augmentative and Alternative Communication*, *17*(3), 99–104.

Fried-Oken, M., Beukelman, D., & Hux, K. (2012). Current and future AAC research considerations for adults with acquired cognitive and communication impairments. *Assistive Technology*, *24*, 56–66.

Gorno-Tempini, M. L., Hillis, A. E., Weintraub, S., Kertesz, A., Mendez, M., Cappa, S. F., . . . Grossman, M. (2011). Classification of primary progressive aphasia and its variants. *Neurology*, *76*(11), 1006–1014.

Glang, A., Ylvisaker, M., Stein, M., Ehlhardt, L., Todis, B., & Tyler, J. (2008). Validated instructional practices: Application to students with traumatic brain injury. *Journal of Head Trauma Rehabilitation*, *23*(4), 243–251.

Harris, J. M., Gall, C., Thompson, J. C., Richardson, A. M., Neary, D., du Plessis, D., . . . Jones, M. (2013). Classification and pathology of primary progressive aphasia. *Neurology*, *81*(21), 1832–1839.

Henry, M. L., & Grasso, S. M. (2018). Assessment of individuals with primary progressive aphasia. *Seminars in Speech and Language, 39*(3), 231–241.

Henry, M. L., Hubbard, H. I., Grasso, S. M., Dial, H. R., Beeson, P. M., Miller, B. L., & Gorno-Tempini, M. L. (2019) Treatment for word retrieval in semantic and logopenic variants of primary progressive aphasia: Immediate and long-term outcomes. *Journal of Speech, Language, and Hearing Research, 62*(8), 2723–2749.

Henry, M. L., Hubbard, H. I., Grasso, S. M., Mandelli, M. L., Wilson, S. M., Sathishkumar, M. T., . . . Gorno-Tempini, M. L. (2018). Retraining speech production and fluency in non-fluent-agrammatic primary progressive aphasia. *Brain, 141*(6), 1799–1814.

Henry, M. L., Meese, M. V., Truong, S., Babiak, M. C., Miller, B. L., & Gorno-Tempini, M. L. (2013a). Treatment for apraxia of speech in nonfluent variant primary progressive aphasia. *Behavioral Neurology, 26*(1–2), 77–88.

Henry, M. L., Rising, K., DeMarco, A. T., Miller, B. L., GornoTempini, M. L., & Beeson, P. M. (2013b). Examining the value of lexical retrieval treatment in primary progressive aphasia: Two positive cases. *Brain and Language, 127*(2), 145–156.

Holland A. L., & Nelson, R. L. (2020). *Counseling in communications disorders: A wellness perspective* (3rd ed.). San Diego, CA: Plural Publishing.

Holland, A. L., Weinberg, P., & Dittelman, J. (2012). How to use apps clinically in the treatment of aphasia. *Seminars in Speech and Language: Adult Focus, 33*(3), 223–233.

Holland, A. L., Fromm, D., & Wozniak, L. (2018). *CADL-3: Communication Activities of Daily Living* (3rd ed.). Austin, TX: Pro-Ed.

Hopper, T., Bourgeois, M., Pimentel, J., Qualls, C. D., Hickey, E., Frymark, T., & Schooling, T. (2013). An evidence-based systematic review on cognitive interventions for individuals with dementia. *American Journal of Speech-Language Pathology, 22*, 126–145.

Jokel, R., Graham, N. L., Rochon, E., & Leonard, C. (2014). Word retrieval therapies in primary progressive aphasia. *Aphasiology, 28*(8/9), 1038–1068.

Jokel, R., & Meltzer, J. (2017) Group intervention for individuals with primary progressive aphasia and their spouses: Who comes first? *Journal of Communication Disorders, 66*, 51–64.

Kagan, A. (1998). Supported conversation for adults with aphasia: Methods and resources for training conversation partners, *Aphasiology, 12*(9), 816–830.

Kagan, A., Simmons-Mackie, N., Rowland, A., Huijbregts, M., Shumway, E., McEwen, S., . . . Sharp, S. (2008). Counting what counts: A framework for capturing real-life outcomes of aphasia intervention. *Aphasiology, 22*(3), 258–280.

Khayum, B., Wieneke, C., Rogalski, E., Robinson, J., & O'Hara, M. (2012). Thinking outside the stroke: Treating primary progressive aphasia (PPA). ASHA SIG 15 *Perspectives on Gerontology, 17*, 37–49.

Kim, E. S., Figeys, M., Hubbard, H. I., & Wilson, C. (2018). The impact of aphasia camp participation on quality of life: A primary progressive aphasia perspective. *Seminars in Speech and Language, 39*(3), 270–283.

Kortte, K. B., & Rogalski E. J. (2013). Behavioural interventions for enhancing life participation in behavioural variant frontotemporal dementia and primary progressive aphasia. *International Review of Psychiatry, 25*(2), 237–245.

Matias-Guiu, J. A., & Garcia-Ramos, R. (2013). Primary progressive aphasia: From syndrome to disease. *Neurologia, 28*(6), 366–374.

Medina, J., & Weintraub, S. (2007). Depression in primary progressive aphasia. *Journal of Geriatric Psychiatry and Neurology, 20*(3), 153–160.

Mesulam, M. M. (1982). Slowly progressive aphasia without generalized dementia. *Annals of Neurology, 11*(6), 592–598.

Mesulam, M. M., Rogalski, E. J., Wieneke, C., Hurley R. S., Geula, C., Bigio, E. H., . . . Weintraub, S (2014). Primary progressive aphasia and the evolving neurology of the language network. *National Review of Neurology, 10*(10), 554–569.

Mesulam, M. M., Weintraub, S., Rogalski, E. J., Wieneke, C., Geula, C., & Bigio, E. (2014). Asymmetry and heterogeneity of Alzheimer's and frontotemporal pathology in primary progressive aphasia. *Brain, 137*(4), 1176–1192.

Mesulam, M. M., Wieneke, C., Thompson, C., Rogalski, E., & Weintraub, S. (2012). Quantitative classification of primary progressive aphasia at early and mild impairment stages. *Brain, 135*(5), 1537–1553.

Mooney, A., Bedrick, S., Noethe, G., Spaulding, S., & Fried-Oken, M. (2018). Mobile technology to support lexical retrieval during activity retell in primary progressive aphasia. *Aphasiology, 32*(6), 666–692.

Mooney, A., Beale, N., & Fried-Oken, M. (2018). Group communication treatment for individuals with PPA and their partners. *Seminars in Speech and Language, 39*(3), 257–269.

Morhardt, D. J., O'Hara, M. C., Zachrich, K., Wieneke, C., & Rogalski, E. J. (2017). Development of a psycho-educational support program for individuals with primary progressive aphasia and their care-partners. *Dementia, 18*(4), 1310–1327.

Morhardt, D., Weintraub, S., Khayum, B., Robinson, J., Medina, J., O'Hara, M., Mesulam, M., & Rogalski, E.J., 2015). The CARE pathway model for dementia: Psychosocial and rehabilitative strategies for care in young-onset dementias. *Psychiatric Clinics of North America*, *38*(2), 333–352.

Pattee, C., Von Berg, S., & Ghezzi, P. (2006). Effects of alternative communication on the communicative effectiveness of an individual with a progressive language disorder. *International Journal of Rehabilitation Research*, *29*(2), 151–153.

Riedl, L., Last, D., Danek, A., & Diehl-Schmid, J. (2014). Long-term follow-up in primary progressive aphasia: Clinical course and health care utilization. *Aphasiology*, *28*(8–9), 981–992.

Rogalski, E. J., & Khayum, B. (2018). A life participation approach to primary progressive aphasia intervention. *Seminars in Speech and Language*, *39*, 284–296.

Rogalski, E. J., Saxon, M., McKenna, H., Wieneke, C., Rademaker A., Corden, M.E., . . . Khayum, B. (2016). Communication bridge: A pilot feasibility study of internet-based speech-language therapy for individuals with progressive aphasia. *Alzheimer's & Dementia: Translational Research & Clinical Interventions*, *2*(4), 213–221.

Rogers, M. A., & Alarcon, N. B. (1998). Dissolution of spoken language in primary progressive aphasia. *Aphasiology*, *12*(7–8), 635–650.

Rogers, M., King, J. M., & Alarcon, N. (2000). Proactive management of primary progressive aphasia In D. Beukelman, K. Yorkston, & J. Reichle (Eds.), *Augmentative and alternative communication for adults with acquired neurologic disorders* (pp. 305–337). Baltimore, MD: Brookes.

Rosenbek, J. C., Lemme, M. L., Ahern, M. B., Harris, E. H., & Wertz, R. T. (1973). A treatment for apraxia of speech in adults. *Journal of Speech and Hearing Disorders*, *38*(4), 462–472.

Simmons-Mackie, N., Kagan, A., Victor, J. C., Carling-Rowland, A., Mok, A., Hoch, J. S., & Streiner, D. L., (2014). The assessment for living with aphasia: Reliability and construct validity. *International Journal of Speech-Language Pathology*, *16*(1), 82–94.

Volkmer, A., Spector, A., Meitanis, V., Warren, J. D., & Beeke, S. (2019). Effects of functional communication interventions for people with primary progressive aphasia and their caregivers: A systematic review *Aging and Mental Health*. https://doi.org/10.1080/136078 63.2019.1617246

Youmans, G. L., Holland, A. L., Munoz, M., & Bourgeois, M. (2005). Script training and automaticity in two individuals with aphasia. *Aphasiology*, *19*, 435–450.

7

LIFE PARTICIPATION FOR PEOPLE WITH DEMENTIA

Natalie F. Douglas and Delainey Smyth

$\mathcal{T}$he Social Imperative charges us to embrace the whole person, including the impairment of language, and in the case of dementia, memory. The charge of the social imperative is too great for us to remain in our silos of comfort. On the one hand, it is necessary to write measurable goals and comply with other regulations that are reimbursable for third party payors, or none of us would have a job. On the other hand, if we only comply with the existing health care system, might we be complicit in keeping this system broken? What does this mean for the people we serve?

None of these issues are easy or simple to solve, but this book is a step in the right direction. In the following chapter, background information about dementia, person-centered care, and life participation will be provided. Next, a summary of evidence-based approaches that may support life participation for someone with dementia will be highlighted. It is easy to forget that people with dementia, just like others in this book, may at some point require hospitalization post dementia diagnosis. Thus, we will discuss three cases across the continuum of care: hospitalization, subsequently skilled nursing, and finally community dwelling. These cases will illustrate the concepts further with measurable goals and resources that current SLPs will hopefully find useful. Concluding remarks will suggest future directions of incorporating the life participation approach to dementia.

Background

Dementia is a public health crisis, and there is likely not one of us who is immune to the tragic sting of this syndrome (World Health Organization [WHO]; 2019). Although the etiologies are many, Alzheimer's disease being the most common, dementia is an umbrella term that encompasses deficits in memory, thinking, executive functioning, visuo-spatial skills, and otherwise, that impact social and/or occupational functioning (National Institute on Aging (NIA); n.d.). These deficits can often lead people with dementia to rely on others for daily care, even for basic activities of daily living such as showering, eating, and going to the bathroom (Prizer & Zimmerman, 2018).

Speech-language pathologists have worked with people with dementia for decades and should be considered leaders when managing the cognitive-communication disorders that ultimately arise for many people living with dementia (ASHA, 2016; Bourgeois, Brush, Douglas, Khayum, & Rogalski, 2016). And although a diagnosis with dementia is devastating, there are many cases of people living successfully with the syndrome, enjoying autonomy and agency even until their last days (Lin & Lewis, 2015; Peoples, Pedersen, & Moestrup, 2018). Returning to the Social Imperative for people with aphasia, there remains such an imperative for people with dementia as well.

A recent randomized controlled trial found that spending just one-hour weekly conversing with someone with dementia about a topic of interest resulted in better health outcomes across the board for people with dementia (Ballard et al., 2018). Similarly, a meta-analysis indicated that models of care that incorporated person-centeredness and strengths-based programming were superior to traditional medical models that only focused on "fixing what is broken" for people with dementia (Kim & Park, 2017). Although a full review of the literature is outside of the scope of this chapter, there is evidence pointing to the benefits of the life participation approach for people with dementia.

Other chapters in this book discuss the A-FROM model where a speech-language pathologist (SLP) working with someone living with aphasia may seek to intervene either directly or indirectly at the level of (a) participation in life situations; (b) personal, identity, attitudes and feelings; (c) language and related impairments; or (d) communication and language environment (Kagan et al., 2008). For people with dementia, SLPs may consider the FROM model that was designed to be a more generic version of this model, designed to capture meaningful outcomes, but without the "aphasia." For instance, people with dementia can live satisfying and happy lives. They have the potential to participate actively in life situations with environmental supports, communication aids and situation specific training. People with dementia also experience a wide array of feelings, issues of identities, and attitudes despite living with cognitive impairment.

Person-Centered Care and Life Participation

The life participation approach to dementia is not a frequently used phrase in the dementia literature. Although the principles are much the same, it is more common to speak about person-centered care for people with dementia. Person-centered care (PCC) for people with dementia is related to life participation as PCC strives to incorporate the values and strengths of the person into the center of care planning. A person-centered clinical method (Levenstein, McCracken McWhinney, Stewart, & Brown, 1986; Brown, Stewart, McCracken, McWhinney, & Levenstein, 1986; Greenhalgh, 2018) has been described as ". . . the sharing of decisions and responsibilities between patients and providers; the strengthening of practitioners' compassion, sensitivity to patients' distress and commitment to respond to patients with empathy in an effort to alleviate suffering . . . " (Liberati, Goril, Moja, Galuppo, Ripamonti, & Scaratti, 2015, p. 46). Nickel, Weinberger and Guze (2018) further describe person-centered care along four principles:

1. People should be treated with dignity, compassion, and respect.
2. People are active partners in all aspects of their care.
3. People should contribute to the development and improvement of healthcare systems.
4. People should be partners in the education of healthcare professionals.

Persons with dementia need PCC and opportunities to participate in the fullest lives they can maintain, despite the loss of cognitive skills. There are many evidence-based approaches to support the personhood, life participation, and cognitive-communication status of people with dementia. Although a review of these treatments in detail is outside the scope of this chapter, some of them will be described briefly below.

Guiding Principles and Evidence-Based Intervention for Dementia Care

Dementia care should be grounded in three main areas—maximizing independent functioning for as long as possible; maintaining quality of life via supported engagement and participation; and emphasizing personal relevance and contextual training (Hickey & Bourgeois, 2018). Here we summarize approaches that can be incorporated into treatment planning to support life participation of people living with dementia.

External Memory Aids

External memory aids are any outside support that may facilitate either memory or communication in someone with dementia (Bourgeois, 1992; Bourgeois, 1993; Bourgeois, Burgio, Shulz, Beach, & Palmer, 1997; Bourgeois, Dijkstra, Burgio, & Allen-Burge, 2001; Bourgeois, 2014). They could take the form of communication wallets with key phrases or personally relevant vocabulary, memory index cards to reduce repetitive questioning, memory books about pleasant topics of conversation or biographical events, or even name tags, to name a few. External memory aids could be provided in simple pen/paper formats, typed up and printed out, or presented electronically through a tablet or other electronic device. External memory aids may be framed to support a home-like environment, and they should always be constructed with a font size large enough for the person with dementia to read and with appropriate contrasting colors (Bourgeois, 1992, 2014; Bourgeois et al., 1997, 2001).

Spaced Retrieval Training

Spaced retrieval training is another evidence-based intervention that can be leveraged to support life participation for someone with dementia. When a person-centered need or desire is identified, a lead question is developed, a response is formulated, and practice intervals with a clinician or care partner are implemented. Timing is increased to the next interval or decreased to the last successful interval based upon client performance (Brush & Camp, 1998b; Benigas, Brush, & Elliot, 2016). For example, a lead question might be, "What do you do when you want to know when lunchtime is?" A response may be, "I look down at my schedule." The process would begin with the person with dementia repeating the target response directly after the clinician or care partner states the answer, and then progress in seconds based on success. Spaced retrieval training is often used in conjunction with external memory aids as a form of training to support external memory aid usage.

Montessori-Based Activities

Montessori principles can be adapted into a philosophy of care designed to support independence, meaningful engagement, and purposeful activities for older adults (Douglas, Brush, & Bourgeois, 2018; Brush, Douglas, & Bourgeois, 2018). Major components include a prepared environment, the engagement of leadership, and trained Montessori care partners. Elders with differing strengths and weaknesses are encouraged to choose activities based on their preferences, and they are also encouraged to engage in uninterrupted blocks of activity time based upon their own desires, not the desires of an institution or family member. Specialized activity materials and freedom of physical movement are also encouraged. Readers are referred to https://www.brushdevelopment.com for more information and trainings about this philosophy of care.

Meaningful engagement involves activities that support independence, choice, and the well-being of people living with dementia. The person with dementia may engage in an activity in different ways, and it is the person with dementia who determines what is meaningful. Sources for determination of what is meaningful and important to the person with dementia may include assessing both past and present interests, leisure activities, prior or current achievements, or comfort items such as a pet, special blanket, or photo.

Intergenerational Programming

There is evidence for the benefits of intergenerational programming for people with dementia (Listokin, 2011; Mahendra & Hopper, 2013). Through service-learning opportunities, volunteers decrease their negative attitudes towards older adults, improve their communication skills, and decrease their fears of communicating with people with dementia (Mahendra & Hopper, 2013; Heuer, Douglas, Burney, & Willer, 2019). Preliminary outcomes point to positive changes in life participation for people with dementia during interactions with undergraduate students when the students were coached to help the person with dementia select and modify activities according to their strengths (Smyth & Douglas, 2019).

Technology

As technology rapidly develops, there are currently several applications that can support people with dementia participating in life (Lorenz, Freddolino, Comas-Herrera, Knapp, & Damant,

2017). There are tools such as "dementia" clocks that serve as an external memory aid for people with dementia, devices for medication management, and video monitoring. GPS location tracking and related devices can also support people with dementia potentially living independently for longer. Picture phones, tools for appliance use monitoring, and wearable cameras also have the potential to support people living with dementia. Additional safety tools include alarms, fall detectors, and water temperature monitors (Lorenz et al., 2017). Tools to support receiving therapy services online and educational programs for care partners are additional helpful technology applications.

It is also possible that in the near future, home care robots and other smart devices may become more accessible, not to replace the human care partner, but to potentially decrease their burden (Astell et al., 2019). For example, "Paro" is a therapeutic, robotic seal that has been shown to decrease stress in both people with dementia and their care partners (Burton, 2013). Research teams are continuing to assess the benefits of virtual reality and simulated presence for people living with dementia as well. A recent randomized controlled trial found that family video messaging presented on a tablet was beneficial in decreasing confusion of people with dementia in the hospital. The family video messaging worked better than a control group who were shown peaceful nature scenes on the tablet (Waszynskia, Milner, Staff, & Molonyd, 2018).

Music

Music can be a way that people, even in severe stages of dementia, can experience pleasure and some level of life participation (Perez-Ros, Cubero-Plazas, Mejias-Serrano, Cunha, & Martinez-Arnau, 2019). Placing headphones on someone with dementia with their preferred music has supported meaningful engagement. The music should be personalized to the person's preferences. Some studies indicate that music that was popular around the time the person with dementia was 15 or 16 years old may be particularly enjoyable, or used as a starting point to assess the person's musical interests (Thomas, Baier, Kosar, Ogarek, Trepman, & Mor, 2017).

Environmental Modifications

Manipulating the environment is a powerful intervention to support communication for people with dementia (van Hoof et al., 2010). The environment should be organized and esthetically pleasing (Douglas et al., 2018). It should provide enticement to engage and also to have dedicated interactive spaces. The environment should provide appropriate cues to support independence and offer materials that are accessible at any time. Considerations include designated areas for socialization, quiet contemplation, reading, and intimacy. The environment should also provide safe and frequent access to the outdoors with real, not children's, objects of interest. It should be uncluttered and well maintained, reflecting peace and tranquility and inviting the person to engage.

The next section will illustrate these practices in more detail through case examples. Each case provides options for assessment and targets for intervention, including possible measurable goals.

Acute Care

It can sometimes be forgotten that people with dementia have health care needs and that hospitalization post dementia diagnosis may be necessary. Unfortunately, people with dementia have poorer outcomes when they are admitted to the hospital than people without dementia (Hermann, Muck, & Nehen, 2015). People with dementia also have less access to rehabilitative services if they have sustained a stroke (Timmons et al., 2015). No matter their cognitive status, people with dementia are still entitled to access to communication. O'Halloran, Worrall, and Hickson (2012) stated it well:

> People need to be able to communicate with their health care providers as effectively as possible to get adequate, appropriate, and timely health care. People with communication disabilities are at risk of being unable to communicate effectively with their health care providers and this can have consequences on their care. (p. S832)

One may receive a referral for someone with dementia in the acute care stages due to a person sustaining increased confusion or someone having difficulty communicating with health care staff. The person may additionally be on a modified diet due to dysphagia. In this case example, Mr. Jones has a primary medical diagnosis of moderate to severe dementia, and he was hospitalized from a skilled nursing facility due to dehydration and a community acquired pneumonia. Mr. Jones participated in meaningful activities throughout his time in the skilled nursing facility. He was often found joking with nurses and interacting with other residents about sports. Unfortunately, his confusion upon entry into the hospital caused the social worker to think that Mr. Jones would need to be moved to a locked memory unit, a more restricted environment than his current one. Thankfully, the team decided to consult with speech-language pathology in hopes that they could help Mr. Jones with cognitive-communication needs.

Assessment

Bourgeois and colleagues recommend "flipping the rehab model" in terms of assessment of people with dementia (Bourgeois et al., 2016). It is important to begin with the end in mind (Kagan & Simmons-Mackie, 2007). For Mr. Jones, some key questions included:

What does Mr. Jones need to be able to do to function optimally in the environment?

What is Mr. Jones' current cognitive-communication status when not in the hospital?

How is he able to consent (or not) for medical procedures?

How is Mr. Jones oriented to who is caring for him and what for?

How is Mr. Jones expressing wants and needs?

Assessment for Mr. Jones included a detailed medication and chart review, an interview with staff, informal assessment, and administration of the *Inpatient Functional Interview: Screening, Assessment, and Intervention* (IFCI-SAI; O'Halloran, Worrall, Toffolo, & Code, 2020). During administration of the IFCI interview portion, it was noted that Mr. Jones was having difficulty communicating needs, including when he needed to use the bathroom and when he needed help adjusting the temperature in the room. With the use of visual supports, Mr. Jones improved his communication skills; however, visual supports needed to be simple and in large, 24-point font. Also, the topic of the Detroit Tigers seemed to help Mr. Jones communicate in a way that was more typical for him, according to his care team at the skilled nursing facility.

Treatment

The implementation of a Health Care Communication Plan (O'Halloran et al., 2020) in the acute phases of illness may involve the following goals and procedures, with an emphasis on training health care providers involved in his care.

1. Mr. Jones will be oriented to place, person, time, and procedure with attention to external memory aids in 8/10 trials.

Procedures for implementation may include using spaced retrieval training to attend to the memory aids, a large print dry erase board, and memory books for common procedures such as x-rays or blood draws. These memory books can be displayed in either electronic or paper/pen forms.

2. Mr. Jones will have access to alternative modes of communication in easily accessible places.

Procedures for implementation may include pen, paper and multiple communication boards in different places in the room. A board to represent yes/no to provide consent for medical procedures (or not) should also be available. A note stating, "Ask me about the Tigers," could also be nearby. Free resources including a medical encounter board and bedside messages board are available at https://widgit-health.com/downloads/for-professionals.htm

Accessible health care for people with dementia requires continuity of care. For example, in the acute care stages of care, it is important to check in with the next point of care. This may be the home health, assisted living, skilled nursing, or outpatient setting. A simple phone call, e-mail, or perhaps more formal communication will facilitate life participation for the person living with dementia as they move out of the hospital setting. For example, the acute care SLP would not have known that Mr. Jones was a jokester or a Tigers fan if not for that simple phone call.

Skilled Nursing Facility

A referral for someone living with dementia in a skilled nursing facility (SNF) setting may occur due to the elder experiencing restlessness, boredom, or repetitive questioning throughout the day. These responsive behaviors may cause significant burden to staff and other elders in the living community.

Assessment

In this particular case, Mrs. Smith was diagnosed with moderate dementia of the Alzheimer's type. On the *Montreal Cognitive Assessment* (MOCA; Nasserdine et al., 2005), she achieved a score of "2." Informal interviewing and other methods of informal assessment as well as "flipping the rehab model" revealed that participation in life situations along with personal identity, attitudes, and feelings were areas for intervention. Beginning with the end in mind, the following questions were asked:

What does Mrs. Smith need to be able to do to function optimally in the SNF environment?

What does Mrs. Smith want to do, and how does she want to spend her days?

Considerations of Mrs. Smith's interests and hobbies should be of utmost importance. The Pioneer Network offers a significant amount of open-access, free resources to implement

person-centered care and these are available here https://www
.pioneernetwork.net/resource-library/. The freely available *Preferences for Everyday Living (PELI*; Van Haitsma, 2019) is another
tool designed to assess the preferences of someone living with
dementia in this setting.

Informal measures should also include a vision and reading
screening, particularly to determine font size for visual cues, a
color perception screening, and the person's ability to perceive
photos or pictures. For example, Mrs. Smith was able to read aloud,
but only when the font was 36-point. Observations of strengths,
interests, participation, responsive behaviors, and unmet needs
should also be completed. Options for standard measures
include the *Functional Linguistic Communication Inventory*
(Bayles & Tomeoda, 1994), *Scales of Cognitive-Communication
Ability for Neurorehabilitation* (Milman & Holland, 2012), and
the *Arizona Battery for Communication Disorders of Demen-
tia-2* (Bayles & Tomoeda 2018).

Assessment tasks also revealed that Mrs. Smith did not enjoy
the typical activities that were happening in the facility. She felt
that she did not have much choice when it was activity time. She
did not want to go to Bingo, and she did not want to go to group
exercise, but she also did not want to stay in her room all day.
What was perceived as restlessness and boredom was actually
Mrs. Smith lacking a functional way to communicate her preferences. Assessment revealed that Mrs. Smith did enjoy reading,
arranging flowers, folding laundry, and chatting with others in
small groups about her life.

Treatment

Skilled speech therapy goals to be implemented in this environment to support access to communication are provided below:

1. Mrs. Smith will attend to a visual reminder to "Please
   enjoy reading a book," in 5/5 trials over three consecutive
   sessions after environmental modifications.
2. Mrs. Smith will attend to a visual reminder to "Please fold
   the laundry" after spaced retrieval training of the lead
   question, "What do you do when you see the clean clothes

in the basket?" Target answer, "Fold the laundry," in 4/5 trials over three consecutive sessions.

3. Mrs. Smith will use a personalized memory book after meals for at least 15 minutes, three times per day, when directed by a staff member.

4. Mrs. Smith will participate in two interactional conversations with staff of at least six conversational turns on identified topics of personal interest after staff takes her to the bathroom during the day.

Part of intervention for a person living with dementia should include a functional maintenance plan after skilled services have been provided. This is a plan that allows staff such as certified nursing assistants, rehabilitation technicians, or activities professionals to guide people with dementia toward activities supporting life participation following skilled intervention from a speech-language pathologist. An example functional maintenance plan could include the following:

Area of Concern—Mrs. Smith demonstrates increased wandering and restlessness throughout the day and often bothers other elders in the community.

Goal—Mrs. Smith will engage in meaningful activity with the support of visual cues and caregiver assistance.

Approaches and Intervention—
1. Mrs. Smith will use a memory book for meaningful conversation three times daily after meals in 5/7 days per week.
2. Mrs. Smith will arrange flowers and place on dining tables before lunch in 3/5 days per week using outlined templates for visual cues.

Community Dwelling Individuals

The majority of people living with dementia reside at home in their community (Lepore, Ferrell, & Wiener, 2017). Home health services may be warranted for multiple reasons including after a recent hospitalization due to a urinary tract infection. In another case-study scenario, Mrs. Foner demonstrates receipt of these services. Orders for cognitive-communicative services were received due to increased confusion resulting in caregiver burden for Mrs. Foner's spouse, Mr. Foner. Mr. Foner was worried that he would have to consider a long-term care placement for Mrs. Foner, and he deeply desired to keep her at home. The home-health team was cautiously optimistic that Mrs. Foner could remain living at home with appropriate skilled speech therapy services.

Assessment

Assessment materials included a combination of interviews, questionnaires, and standardized measures including a home safety checklist. Mrs. Foner has a history significant for mild vascular dementia. Assessment procedures included the formal test of the *Scales of Cognitive and Communicative Ability for Neurorehabilitation* (Milman & Holland, 2012) that revealed difficulties in memory, orientation, and problem solving. The *Environment and Communication Assessment Toolkit for Dementia* (Brush, Calkins, Bruce, & Sanford, 2012) was also administered and revealed numerous avenues for intervention, such as the need for visual supports and lighting suggestions. It also revealed that Mrs. Foner reads aloud in a 16-point font. Tools to support a "dementia" friendly environment are freely available from the Social Care Institute of Excellence based out of the United Kingdom (https://www.scie.org.uk/dementia/supporting-people-with-dementia/dementia-friendly-environments/). The *Life Interests and Values (LIV) Cards* (Haley, Womack, Helm-Estabrooks, Lovette, & Goff, 2013) was also administered to Mr. and Mrs. Foner to further assess opportunities for life participation. Results of this assessment revealed opportunities for intervention at the level of participation in life situations, communication and the language environment, and personal, identity, attitudes, and feelings. The SLP concluded that part of Mrs. Foner's frustration was due to the changing roles in her marriage. Mrs. Foner desired to interact with her family and not feel "like a patient" all the time. These feelings contributed to her withdrawal from Mr. Foner and her feelings of restlessness, upset, and confusion.

Treatment

Skilled speech therapy goals for Mrs. Foner and her care partner are provided and described below:

1. Mr. Foner will conduct three optimal environmental modifications to support orientation and communication for his wife, Mrs. Foner, in the home setting over a period of two weeks.

Target environmental modifications may include contrasting colors for plates and tablecloths and labeling of key appliances in a 16-point font. The care partner could be instructed to place two pieces of preferential artwork to support finding the way from the kitchen to the bedroom and from the bathroom to the living room. The final environmental modification could be to move furniture to promote an open view of the outside, and easy, safe access to the garden area.

2. Mrs. Foner will FaceTime two grandchildren two times weekly with the use of visual supports on their simplified iPad over a period of two weeks.

Key pieces for implementation include simplifying the number and look of applications on the iPad home screen, creating a visual cue with appropriate font and contrast concerning how to operate FaceTime, and implementing spaced-retrieval training to support attention to visual cues for the FaceTime call. Other potential goals may include the following:

3. Mrs. Foner will engage in purposeful activity between meals, including writing a positive message to granddaughters and folding laundry (activities based on interests) for at least 15 minutes.
4. Mr. Foner will connect to a support group and enroll in respite care 2× monthly for at least two hours.

5. Mr. Foner will continue spaced retrieval training for the repeated question "Where's Sally?" to refer to the external memory aid that says, "Sally will visit very soon" whenever the question is asked by Mrs. Foner throughout the day.

6. Mr. Foner will address five safety concerns per the home safety checklist to optimize the environment for safety and communication.

Care Partner Training Considerations

A discussion about the implementation of the life participation approach for people with dementia is not complete without revisiting the role of care partners. Research has shown the importance of incorporating adult learning principles such as focus upon the need to know, self-concept, the learner's experiences, readiness to learn, orientation to learning, and motivation when considering training care partners (Hickey & Bourgeois, 2018). Ideally, training in a cognitive-communication strategy for a care partner is based off of a problem that the care partner has identified and that they are internally motivated to solve. For example, if repetitive questioning is a burdensome enough issue, the care partner may be open to trying multiple strategies to attempt to help the situation. Consider using short, in-the-moment coaching sessions in lieu of longer didactic sessions (Troyna & Douglas, 2018). For example, a care partner might receive more benefit from an in the moment coaching session of communication strategies during meal time than attending a generalized workshop about communication strategies for people with dementia during meal time.

Specific communication strategies for care partners are valuable, including using short and simple sentences, speaking slowly, asking one question or giving one instruction at a time, eliminating distractions, avoiding interruption, allowing plenty of time for responding, using yes/no rather than open-ended questions, encouraging circumlocution during word finding problems, and repeating/rephrasing messages (Bourgeois, 2014). The FOCUSED care partner training program suggests that care partners speak **face-to-face** about **functional** topics with the person with dementia. It strongly suggests that care partners should **orient** the person with dementia to the conversation topic by providing **continuity** in the conversation about **concrete** topics. Care partners may **"unstick"** any communication blocks with cues, such as visual supports. They should **structure** the conversation in a way that offers yes/no as well as and/or choice questions. Encouraging interaction and an **exchange** of ideas is also part of the FOCUSED care partner training program. Finally, the last part of this training program suggests that communication should be **direct** and made up of short, simple sentences to support participation for the person with dementia (Ripich, Wykle, & Niles, 1995).

There are many free modules that include video examples of common difficulties experienced by care partners from the University of California, Los Angeles (available at https://www.uclahealth.org/dementia/caregiver-education-videos). Although there are benefits to providing care for someone with dementia, full-time care partners are at significant risk for caregiver burden (Cheng, 2017). Care partners should be encouraged to care for themselves and take advantage of respite and other care partner-based interventions (Walter & Pinquart, 2019).

Summary and Future Directions

People with dementia can benefit from speech-language pathology services to support life participation, even in the acute phases of illness. Even though dementia is progressive, intervention can help maintain the person's cognitive-communication skills. Elements of the FROM model, such as participation in life situations, communication and the language environment, personal identity, attitudes, and feelings are excellent starting points for treatment planning.

Life participation for people with dementia requires the SLP to be a collaborative member or leader of the interprofessional/interdisciplinary team (Lichtenstein et al., 2015). Future considerations for SLPs fully supporting people with dementia includes engaging with policy makers and administrators about their key role with this population. This involves communicating in ways that may be outside the traditional training of a clinician and may include constructing policy briefs, participating in quality improvement or quality assurance/performance improvement initiatives, or connecting to the organizational vision and mission to advocate for service provision. The Social Imperative applies to those living with dementia as well as aphasia.

References

American Speech-Language-Hearing Association. (2016). *Scope of practice in speech-language pathology* [Scope of practice]. Retrieved from http://www.asha.org/policy/

Astell, A. J., Bourains, N., Hoey, J., Lindauer, A., Mihailidis, A., Nugent, C., & Robillard, J. (2019). Technology and dementia: The future is now. *Dementia and Geriatric Cognitive Disorders, 47,* 131–139. https://doi.org/10.1159/000497800

Ballard, C., Corbett, A., Orrell, M., Williams, G., Moniz-Cook, E., Romeo, R., Woods, B., . . . Fossey, J. (2018). Impact of person-centred care training and person-centred activities on quality of life, agitation, and antipsychotic use in people with dementia living in nursing homes: A cluster-randomised controlled trial. *PLOS Medicine, 15*(2), 1–18. https://doi.org/10.1371/journal.pmed.1002500

Bayles, K. A., & Tomoeda, C. K. (1994). *Functional Linguistic Communication Inventory.* Austin, TX: Pro-Ed.

Bayles, K. A., & Tomoeda, C. K. (2018). *Arizona Battery for Cognitive Communication Disorders* (2nd ed.). Austin, TX: Pro-Ed.

Benigas, J., Brush, J., & Elliot, G. (2016). *Spaced retrieval step by step: An evidence-based memory intervention.* Health Professions Press.

Bourgeois, M. S. (1992). Evaluating memory wallets in conversations with persons with dementia. *Journal of Speech and Hearing Research, 35,* 1344–1357. https://doi.org/10.1044/jshr.3506.1344

Bourgeois, M. S. (1993). Effects of memory aids on the dyadic conversations of individuals with dementia. *Journal of Applied Behavior Analysis, 26,* 77–87. https://doi.org/10.1901%2Fjaba.1993.26-77

Bourgeois, M. S. (2014). *Memory books and other graphic cueing systems: Practical communication and memory aids for adults with dementia.* Towson, MD: Health Professions Press.

Bourgeois, M., Brush, J., Douglas, N. F., Khayum, B., & Rogalski, E. (2016). Will you still need me when I'm 64, or 84, or 104? The importance of SLPs in promoting the quality of life of aging adults in the U.S. into the future. *Seminars in Speech and Language, 37(3),* 185–200. https://doi.org/10.1055/s-0036-1583544

Bourgeois, M. S., Burgio, L. D., Shulz, R., Beach, S., & Palmer, B. (1997). Modifying repetitive verbalizations of community-dwelling residents with AD. *The Gerontologist, 37,* 30–39. https://doi.org/10.1093/geront/37.1.30

Bourgeois, M. S., Dijkstra, K., Burgio, L., & Allen-Burge, R. (2001). Memory aids as an augmentative and alternative communication strategy for nursing home residents with dementia. *Augmentative and Alternative Communication, 17,* 196–210. https://doi.org/10.1080/714043383

Brown, J., Stewart, M., McCracken, E., McWhinney, I. R., & Levenstein, J. (1986). The patient-centered clinical method. Definition and application, *Family Practice, 3*(2), 75–79. https://doi.org/10.1093/fampra/3.2.75

Brush, J., Calkins, M., Bruce, C., & Sanford, J. (2012). *Environmental and communication assessment toolkit for dementia care.* Towson, MD: Health Professions Press.

Brush, J. A., & Camp, C. J. (1998). Using spaced retrieval as an intervention during speech-language therapy. *Clinical Gerontologist, 19*(1), 51–64. https://doi.org/10.1300/J018v19n01_05

Brush, J., Douglas, N. F., & Bourgeois, M. (2018). Implementation of the Montessori philosophy in assisted living: positive outcomes and challenges. *The Journal of Nursing Home Research Sciences, 4,* 64–70.

Burton, A. (2013). Dolphins, dogs and robot seals for the treatment of neurological disease. *Lancet Neurology, 12*(9), 851–852. https://doi.org/10.1016/S1474-4422(13)70206-0

Cheng, S-T. (2017). Dementia caregiver burden: a research update and critical analysis. *Current Psychiatry Reports, 19*(9), 64. https://doi.org/10.1007/s11920-017-0818-2

Douglas, N. F., Brush, J., & Bourgeois, M. (2018). Person-centered, skilled services using a Montessori approach for persons with dementia. *Seminars in Speech and Language, 39*(3), 223–230. https://doi.org/10.1055/s-0038-1660781

Haley, K. L., Womack, J., Helm-Estabrooks, N., Lovette, B., & Goff, R. (2013). Supporting autonomy in persons with aphasia: Use of the life interests and values cards. *Topics in Stroke Rehabilitation, 20*(1), 22–35. https://doi.org/10.1310/tsr2001-22

Hermann, D. M., Muck, S., Nehen, H. G. (2015). Supporting dementia patients in hospital environments: Health related risks, needs and dedicated structures for patient care. *European Journal of Neurology, 22*(2), 239–245. https://doi.org/10.1111/ene.12530

Heuer, S., Douglas, N. F., Burney, T., & Willer, R. (2019). Service-learning with older adults in care communities: Measures of attitude shifts in undergraduate students. *Gerontology & Geriatrics Education.* https://doi.org/10.1080/02701960.2019.1596087

Hickey, E. M., & Bourgeois, M. (2018). *Dementia: Person-centered assessment and intervention* (2nd ed.). New York, NY: Routledge.

Greenhalgh, T. (2018). *How to implement evidence-based healthcare.* Hoboken, NJ: Wiley.

Kagan, A., & Simmons-Mackie, N. (2007). Beginning with the end: Outcome-driven assessment and intervention with life participation in mind. *Topics in Language Disorders, 27*(4), 309–317. https://doi.org/10.1097/01.tld.0000299885.39488.bf

Kagan, A., Simmons-Mackie, N., Rowland, A., Huijbregts, M., Shumway, E., McEwen, S., Threats, T., . . . Sharp, S. (2008). Counting what counts: A framework for capturing real-life outcomes of aphasia intervention. *Aphasiology, 3,* 258–280. https://doi.org/10.1080/02687030701282595

Kim, S. K., & Park, M. (2017). Effectiveness of person-centered care on people with dementia: A systematic review and meta-analysis. *Clinical Interventions in Aging, 12,* 381–387. https://doi.org/10.2147/CIA.S117637

Lepore, M., Ferrell, A., & Wiener, J. M. (2017). *Living arrangements for people with Alzheimer's disease and related dementias: Implications for services and supports.* National Alzheimer's Project Act. Retrieved from https://aspe.hhs.gov/system/files/pdf/257966/LivingArran.pdf

Levenstein, J. H., McCracken, E. C., McWhinney, I. R., Stewart, M. A., & Brown, J. B. (1986). The patient-centered clinical method. A model for the doctor-patient interaction in family medicine. *Family Practice, 3*(1), 24–30. https://doi.org/10.1093/fampra/3.1.24

Liberati, E. G., Goril, M., Moja, L., Galuppo, L., Ripamonti, S., & Scaratti, G. (2015). Exploring the practice of patient-centered care: The role of ethnography and reflexivity. *Social Science Medicine, 133,* 45–52. https://doi.org/10.1016/j.socscimed.2015.03.050

Lichtestein, B. J., Reuben, D. B., Karlamangla, A. S., Han, W., Roth, C. P., & Wegner, N. S. (2015). Effect of physician delegation to other healthcare providers on the quality of care for geriatric conditions. *Journal of the American Geriatrics Society, 63,* 2164–2170. https://doi.org/10.1111/jgs.13654

Lin, S. Y., & Lewis, F. M. (2015). Dementia friendly, dementia capable, and dementia positive: Concepts to prepare for the future. *The Gerontologist, 55*(2), 237–244. https://doi.org/10.1093/geront/gnu122

Listokin, J. (2011). Project N.O.I.S.E.E: intergenerational laughter, squeals and giggles. *Journal of Intergenerational Relationships, 9*(4), 476–480. https://doi.org/10.1080/15350770.2011.619415

Lorenz, K., Freddolino, P.P., Comas-Herrera, A., Knapp, M., & Damant, J. (2017). Technology-based tools for people with dementia and carers: mapping technology on the dementia care pathway. *Dementia*, *18*(2), 725–741. https://doi.org/10.1177/1471301217691617

Mahendra, N., & Hopper, T. (2013). Dementia and related cognitive disorders. In I. Papathanasiou, P. Coppens, & C. Potagas (Eds.), *Aphasia and related neurogenic communication disorders* (pp. 397–430). Burlington, MA: Jones & Bartlett Learning.

Milman, L., & Holland, A. (2012). *Scales of cognitive and communicative ability for neurorehabilitation*. Austin, TX: Pro-Ed.

Nasreddine, Z. S., Phillips, N. A., Bedrian, V., Charbonneau, S., Whitehead, V., Collin, I., . . . Chertkow, H. (2005). The Montreal Cognitive Assessment, MoCA: A brief screening tool for mild cognitive impairment. *Journal of the American Geriatric Society*, *53*(4), 695–699. https://doi.org/10.1111/j.1532-5415.2005.53221.x

National Institute on Aging. (n.d.). *What is dementia? Symptoms, types, and diagnosis*. Retrieved from https://www.nia.nih.gov/health/what-dementia-symptoms-types-and-diagnosis

Nickel, W. K., Weinberger, S. E., & Guze, P. A. (2018). Principles for patient and family partnership in care: An American college of physicians position paper, *Annals of Internal Medicine*, *169*(11), 796–799. https://doi.org/10.7326/M18-0018

O'Halloran, R., Worrall, L., & Hickson, L. (2012). Environmental factors that influence communication for patients with a communication disability in acute hospital stroke units: A qualitative metasynthesis. *Archives of Physical Medicine and Rehabilitation*, *93*(1), S78–S84. https://doi.org/10.1111/j.1460-6984.2011.00077

O'Halloran, R., Worrall, L., Toffolo, D., & Code, C. (2020). *Inpatient functional communication interview: Screening, assessment, and intervention*. San Diego, CA: Plural Publishing.

Peoples, H., Pedersen, L. F., & Moestrup, L. (2018). Creating a meaningful everyday life: Perceptions of relatives of people with dementia and healthcare relatives in the context of a Danish dementia village. *Dementia*. https://doi.org/10.1177/1471301218820480

Pérez-Ros, P., Cubero-Plazas, L., Mejías-Serrano, T., Cunha, C., & Martínez-Arnau, F. M. (2019). Preferred music listening intervention in nursing home residents with cognitive impairment: A randomized intervention study. *Journal of Alzheimer's Disease*, *70*(2) , 433-442. https://doi.org/10.3233/JAD-190361

Prizer, L. P., & Zimmerman, S. (2018). Progressive support for activities of daily living for persons with dementia. *The Gerontologist*, *18*(58, Suppl. 1), S84–S87. https://doi.org/10.1093/geront/gnx103

Ripich, D., Wykle, M., & Niles, S. (1995). The FOCUSED program: A communication skills training program helps nursing assistants to give better care to patients with Alzheimer's disease. *Geriatric Nursing, 16*(1), 15–19. https://doi.org/10.1016/S0197-4572(05)80073-4

Smyth, D., & Douglas, N. F. (2019, November). *Undergraduate student ability to support engagement of residents with dementia: Does coaching matter?* Paper presented at the Annual Convention of the Speech-Language-Hearing Association, Orlando, FL.

Thomas, K. S., Baier, R., Kosar, C., Ogarek, J., Trepman, A., & Mor, V. (2017). Individualized music program is associated with improved outcomes for U.S. nursing home residents with dementia. *The American Journal of Geriatric Psychiatry, 25*(9), 931–938. https://doi.org/10.1016/j.jagp.2017.04.008

Timmons, S., Manning, E., Barrett, A., Brady, N. M., Browne, V., O'Shea, E., . . . Linehan, J. (2015). Dementia in older people admitted to hospital: A regional multi-hospital observational study of prevalence, associations and case recognition. *Age & Ageing, 44*(6), 993–999. https://doi.org/10.1093/ageing/afv131

Troyna, A., & Douglas, N. F. (2018, November). *Positive behavior changes in certified nursing assistants after facilitative coaching intervention.* Paper presented at the Annual Convention of the American Speech-Language-Hearing Association, Boston, MA.

Van Haitsma, K. (2019). This work is licensed under the Creative Commons Attribution–NoDerivatives 4.0 International License. Based on a work at https://preferencebasedliving.com/ To view a copy of this license, visit http://creativecommons.org/licenses/by-nd/4.0/

van Hoof, J., Hort, K. S., van Waarde, H., & Blom, M. M. (2010). Environmental interventions and the design of homes for older adults with dementia: An overview. *American Journal of Alzheimer's Disease and Other Dementias, 25*(3), 202–232. https://doi.org/10.1177/1533317509358885

Walter, E., & Pinquart, M. (2019). How effective are dementia caregiver interventions: An update and comprehensive meta-analysis. *The Gerontologist.* https://doi.org/10.1093/geront/gnz118

Waszynskia, C. M., Milner, K. A., Staff, I., & Molonyd, S. L. (2018). Using simulated family presence to decrease agitation in older hospitalized delirious patients: A randomized controlled trial. *International Journal of Nursing Studies, 77,* 154–161. https://doi.org/10.1016/j.ijnurstu.2017.09.018

World Health Organization (WHO). (2019, September 19). *Dementia.* Retrieved from https://www.who.int/mediacentre/factsheets/fs362/en/

8

THE LIFE PARTICIPATION APPROACH AND SOCIAL REINTEGRATION AFTER TRAUMATIC BRAIN INJURY

Peter Meulenbroek and Louise C. Keegan

Introduction

Communication disorders after traumatic brain injury (TBI) result from a constellation of cognitive and social communication deficits. Cognitive deficits such as memory, attention, awareness, or problem solving can result in communication difficulties in TBI.

Other aspects of impaired cognition in individuals with TBI may be inherently social, such as recognition of emotion or theory of mind. Social and cognitive deficits often result in reduced social participation and meaningful engagement with others. The Life Participation Approach to Aphasia (LPAA) (LPAA Project Group, 2000) easily maps onto the tenets of communication treatment in TBI championed by Ylvisaker, Feeney, and Urbanczyk (1993) and later by Togher, Hand, and Code (1996), Turkstra, McDonald, and DePompei (2001), and Kennedy and Coelho (2005). These researchers all stress modifying the contextually relevant aspects of life and focusing on meaningful social interaction as fundamental to treatment.

The LPAA is both a philosophy and a framework for looking at the clinical interaction of speech-language pathologists (SLPs) and their clients. In this chapter, we will focus on assessment of TBI using the Aphasia: Framework for Outcome Measurement (A-FROM) (Kagan et al., 2008). This chapter is designed to mirror the A-FROM in two sections. The first section addresses the nature of impairments related to communication. The second section addresses the other three components of the A-FROM: (a) the communication environment, (b) personal identity attitudes and feelings, and (c) participation in life events. These three components are so interrelated that separating their content was felt not to reflect accurately upon clinical practice. Practical suggestions for assessment of these aspects of the communication and social life of the individual with TBI will be provided throughout.

Enhanced social participation is the ultimate goal of communication intervention and it is directly influenced by the abilities, identity, and environment of the individual (Meulenbroek et al., 2019). The metric of therapeutic success is highly individualistic, and may differ relative to factors of ability, environment, and identity. Because of the interplay between the environment and the individual this chapter views environmental variables through a client-focused lens. To support this approach, this chapter incorporates Centeredness Theory, a model of social well-being, to assist with guiding the clinical interview and establishing personal goals. Centeredness Theory uses a schematic framework of identity consistent with the treatment principles of the LPAA and Ylvisaker's work (Bloch-Jorgensen et al., 2018; Kagan & Simmons-Mackie, 2007; Ylvisaker & Feeney, 2000). To summarize, the approach advocated for in this chapter is relevant to SLPs who wish to practice in a manner that is committed to person-centered planning and emphasizes the context, routines, and supports of their clients.

The Nature of Impairment in Traumatic Brain Injury

TBI is characterized by the physical head trauma and disruption in consciousness. The frontoventral and temporal regions of the cortices are most often affected by TBI (McAllister, 1992). These areas subserve many aspects of working memory (executive functioning) and social cognition (Adolphs, 2009). Diffuse brain damage is also associated with TBI, causing unpredictable physical effects such as headaches, pain, sensory perception difficulties, vestibular issues, motor speech difficulties, and changes to voice and resonance. Emotional sequelae of a TBI can include anxiety, stress, depression, anger, frustration, as well as emotional lability. The emotional and physical difficulties have a direct relationship to the individual's sense of self and the ability to communicate one's own personal identity and attitudes.

Cognitive-Communication Difficulties

Cognitive-communication difficulties are distinct from language-specific difficulties, manifesting as problems with competent language use in social contexts (e.g., listening, speaking, reading, writing, conversation, and social interaction). Executive dysfunction usually includes difficulty with self-awareness, goal setting, planning and organizing, initiating, inhibiting behaviors, self-monitoring, self-regulation, and problem solving. Other cognitive difficulties associated with TBI include slower cognitive processing and formulation, distractibility, problems multitasking, memory difficulties, and impaired judgment (Constantinidou, Wertheimer, Tsanadis, Evans, & Paul, 2012; Dean & Sterr, 2013).

Cognitive difficulties can impact communication in a variety of ways. Fatigue may result in a lack of enthusiasm or energy for communication exchanges, or attention difficulties may increase comprehension problems. Self-perception of cognitive/social ability is also commonly impaired after TBI (Crosson et al., 1989). Because of self-perception difficulties, individuals with TBI may not be aware of how others interpret their responses (theory of mind) and they may have difficulty recognizing or using social cues. Awareness of their own deficits may impact their impression of their own abilities and the communicative competence others perceive (McDonald, Honan, Kelly, Byom, & Rushby, 2014).

Apathy after TBI can result in poor initiation and development of, and adherence to, personal goals (Gray, Shepherd, McKinlay, Robertson, & Pentland, 1994). Apathy can be reactive to psychological stress or an organic neurobehavioral disorder associated with TBI. Cognitive factors such as attention or executive functions, as well as affective factors such as negative mood, can contribute to the fatigue experienced after TBI (Beaulieu-Bonneau & Morin, 2012; Worthington & Wood, 2018). Motivational variables (food, socialization, etc.) can change following TBI, and aspects related to personal identity may affect motivation in persons with good awareness of their deficits. Someone who once enjoyed going out for dinner before the TBI might consider the environment to be too distracting and overwhelming after their injury.

Cognitive communication deficits can result in functional social communication deficits. For example, difficulty with memory may result in a conversation partner perceiving the person with TBI as being less competent. Aspects of flexibility, abstraction, and adaptation to new rules are also essential skills in face-to-face communication. Such social communication problems arise secondary to supporting cognitive abilities rather than to social cognition directly (Turkstra et al., 2017).

Social Communication and Social Cognition

Social communication is the set of skills that allow an individual to achieve relevant social goals across contexts (Byom et al., in press). Some communication difficulties after TBI are inherently social, impacting the core constructs associated with socialization (Turkstra, 2008; Turkstra et al., 2017). These include recognizing emotions in others or the ability to make efficient and appropriate inferences about other people's thoughts and feelings.

Social cognition refers to a set of perceptual processes related to social cues from the self and others. Social cognition enables interpretation and understanding of one's own and other's emotions, beliefs, and behaviors, and generating responses to these inferences to guide social behavior (Allain, Togher, & Azouvi, 2018). Social cognition embraces three core concepts: (a) emotional perception, (b) social reasoning (inference), (c) and theory of mind (Adolphs, 2009).

Clinical Relevance

Similar to aphasia assessment, many TBI assessment tools focus on identifying the nature of the *impairment*, rather than focusing on its effects on everyday living. Concomitant and related physical, cognitive, social, and emotional difficulties in TBI mean that these assessments examine skills in isolation, in a therapy room, with the resulting performance often not being representative of the performance in natural social settings. Additionally, many treatment methods focus on "teaching to the test" and completing drills that enhance performance on skills such as generative naming, word finding, narrative memory, and so forth.

In 2014, an international group of researchers and clinicians (known as INCOG; Togher et al., 2014) published clinical practice guidelines for cognitive rehabilitation following TBI. There was some evidence that drill-based practice of skills, using strategies that target memory and attention difficulties (e.g., spaced retrieval training and errorless learning) were beneficial. Nevertheless, these researchers stressed that the environmental influences on cognition and communication are highly relevant to clinical intervention. Focusing assessment and treatment on isolated components of language, cognition, and communication may neglect to acknowledge the complexity of these interconnected skills. This underscores the relevance of the LPAA framework in treating persons with TBI.

Initial Interview and Encounters with the Person with Traumatic Brain Injury

To adequately provide services to persons with TBI, it is necessary to understand both the individual, as well as the nature of their deficits. Success in navigating home, work, and social life informs subjective well-being (Diener et al., 2010). So, successful living with TBI might be considered to be satisfaction with self-performance in home, work, and social life. Different environments and contexts require different social conventions. The person with TBI may or may not be aware of social schemas, or their cognitive communication and social cognition deficits may impact execution of those conventions. Ylvisaker and Feeney (2000) illustrate how the schema concept can be used to grasp how a person with TBI assumes different social roles. According to Young (1994), schemas are thoughts that encompass a person's beliefs, experiences, and generalizations about the self, others, and the future. These beliefs inform how we communicate in specific life domains, as well as the culturally appropriate social rules we choose to follow. SLPs can better understand how to shape treatment by understanding schema awareness in persons with TBI.

Bloch-Jorgensen and colleagues (2018) created a social schema model of well-being called Centeredness Theory. Centeredness Theory conceptualizes well-being as a balance between the core life domains of (1) Work, (2) Family, (3), Relationships, and (4) Community (Figure 8–1). Identity lies at the center of and informs all of these social schemas. When viewed as a Venn diagram, Centeredness Theory looks much like the A-FROM and illustrates these essential life factors visually, allowing the SLP to guide an interview with a picture exploring the communication and cognitive demands of everyday life and aspirations to participate in life. The following describes how to use a *Centeredness Theory Interview* to identify life aspects that are important to the client with TBI and examine how they interact with and perceive their environment.

Identity, or *self*, as in the center of Figure 8–1, is a representation of who we are and what we aspire to be. Identity requires the cooperation of other individuals in order to flourish.

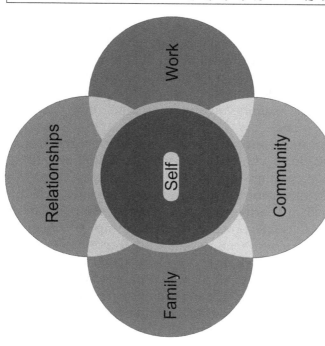

SLP: *The areas on this diagram show aspects of your life that I would like to know more about. When you speak to others the relationships you have with them are important and you share a little bit of yourself in your voice when speaking with family members or people you work with. However, the way you speak at home is different than work.*

Let's use this diagram to talk about what is important to you. All these circles are the same size, but your community life might be smaller (less important) than your family life to you.

Tell me how you wish to communicate in these areas of your life and how important they are to you personally.

Figure 8–1. Centeredness Theory is a model of well-being that incorporates four life domains with the self at the center. We suggest using this approach as a way to structure a client interview for social communication goal development. Adapted from Bloch-Jorgensen, Cilione, Yeung, and Gatt (2018). Centeredness Theory: Understanding and measuring well-being across core life domains. *Frontiers in Psychology, 9,* 610. [This was published under a Creative Commons attribution license (known as a "CC–BY" license, see http://creativecommons.org/licenses/by/4.0/).]

Identity is also dynamic and changes throughout a lifetime, especially if dealing with a traumatic occurrence or a health-related event. A person's identity also contains group identities, with engagement and communication as a constant process in its construction (Eckert, 2000). Acquiring a TBI immediately triggers a shift in identity to one who has experienced/survived a traumatic incident. The sequelae of TBI often result in significant additional identity changes due to difficulties fulfilling previously established life roles. Thus, after TBI one must renegotiate and reconstruct a sense of self, both personally and in concert with others. Social communication difficulties may impede the process of reconstructing identity (Ownsworth, 2014).

The idea that renegotiation of identity is an essential part of life participation after TBI has been well explored in the literature (Keegan, Togher, Murdock, & Hendry, 2017; MacQueen, Fisher, & Williams, 2018). Ylvisaker & Feeney (2000) highlight how negative identities can be self-sustaining, especially when awareness difficulties, negative behavioral responses, and strained relationships are involved. Conversely, research has demonstrated how possessing a positive identity can play a large role in the success of TBI rehabilitation (Keegan et al., 2017; Ownsworth, 2014). Therefore, clinicians should support positive identity development, beginning by selecting interview techniques and assessment measures that examine quality of life and allow clients to assert their own goals.

Motivational interviewing is an interview approach recommended for individuals with brain injury (Miller & Rollnick, 2013). Motivational interviewing supports an individual's autonomy by adopting a nonconfrontational, conversational, eliciting style that is consistent with a "partnership or companionship" relationship rather than an "expert-recipient" relationship. The clinician should respect the client's autonomy and freedom of choice (and its consequences) while recognizing that the client has the power to enact change. Motivational interviewing involves engaging in active listening, making a deliberate effort to withhold judgment, and acknowledging the information and feelings that the person with TBI is communicating. It is imperative to support the person's narrative (Miller & Rollnick, 2013). Lundahl and colleagues (2019) summarize these techniques using the acronym OARS: (a) Open questions; (b) Affirmation of clients' self-efficacy and support; (c) Reflections of clients' thoughts, desires, abilities, reasons, needs, and commitments; and (d) Summaries of the client's history to promote consideration of change. Motivational interviewing approaches are particularly useful for engaging in client-centered goal development.

A *Centeredness Theory Interview* using this approach can focus on the four main life domains of the individual with TBI: Work, Family, Relationship, and Community. Probes seeking how the client relates to others, what they value, and what goals they would like to have for better communication, allows the clinician to establish how an individual's identity influences how they communicate in each of these domains, and forms the basis of a coaching-based intervention (Kennedy, 2017; Ylvisaker, 2006).

Goal Attainment Scaling (GAS) is a method that has recently gained popularity in targeting and working toward collaborative client-centered goal setting (Turner-Stokes, Williams, & Johnson, 2009). GAS is an ecologically valid means of targeting changes in social communication impairments after TBI (Keegan, Murdock, Suger, & Togher, 2019) and enables the client to self-monitor progress. Client motivation and positive identity development are facilitated when clinicians support clients in communicating their aims, and frame goals as targets serving as steps in meeting these aims (Keegan et al., 2019). Figure 8–2 outlines a suggested format of a scaled goal. When SLPs and clients frame goals in a positive light, SLPs can emphasize improvement and progress rather than disability and difficulty supporting a positive identity. Figure 8–2 highlights how goals can be contextualized relative to the LPAA framework using the Rehabilitation Treatment Specification System (Turkstra, Norman, Whyte, Dijkers, & Hart, 2016), in which the clinician documents therapeutic ingredients. A single goal may map to multiple areas of the LPAA framework.

Work

The largest personal cost after TBI is often described as social isolation (Dijkers, 2004). For most adults, work is a major social outlet and a defining characteristic of how they conceptualize themselves in relation to society. A consistent finding is that work return occurs in only approximately 40% of TBI survivors,

Assessment Area	Client Aims	Targets (scaled goals)	Ingredients	Score
Participation in life situations				
Personal identity, attitudes & feelings				
Communication environment				
Communication impairments				←

Goal Attainment Scale

Much more progress than expected	2
Somewhat more progress than expected	1
Expected progress	0
Starting point (level of functioning when goal is established)	-1
Decline in level of functioning	-2

Figure 8–2. Goal Attainment Scaling can be applied to life participation-themed goals focused on the individuals' perceptions about their work, family, relationship, and community participation. The clients' aims can be used for the clinician to develop targets and identify effective treatment ingredients. Progress can be tracked over an established period of time, then compared with baseline performance (value of −1 in Goal Attainment Scaling).

at both 1- and 5-years post injury (Hart et al., 2019). Although satisfaction derived from work and vocational activities is dependent upon subjective individual perceptions, Western society highly values paid employment. Consideration of the life stage and age of the individual at the time of injury factors into the subjective desire to work (Dikmen, Temkin, Machamer, & Holubkov, 1994). Physical, cognitive, and somatic factors all contribute to difficulty with return to work. Deficits in social communication and executive functioning after TBI have also been related to reduced participation in social/vocational outcomes (Meulenbroek & Turkstra, 2016). To deal with the multitude of workplace factors, the SLP needs to take into account: (1) job responsibilities, (2) client's skills and abilities, and (3) the workplace environment (i.e., work culture, physical environment, employer characteristics, etc.).

The *Centeredness Theory Interview* can be used to assess job responsibilities. The SLP can probe for relevant factors related to workplace communication by conducting a workplace task analysis or job analysis (Prien, Goodstein, Goodstein, & Gamble, 2009). This analysis, a set of questions about the nature of the job requirements, environment, and social climate (Prien et. al., 2009), can be completed with the person who has sustained a TBI during the *Centeredness Theory Interview*, or separately with a colleague or employer. These demands are weighed with the impairments and strengths of the individual with TBI as well as with the individual's aspirations regarding work return. Figure 8–3 shows a basic workplace task analysis worksheet that the SLP can fill in with areas of interest regarding communication abilities based on initial assessment. Colleagues from work often provide more explicit information on the nature of tasks related to a job than do the employer or supervisor (Meulenbroek, Bowers, & Turkstra, 2016), and comparing multiple perspectives can provide a more holistic picture of functioning in the setting.

Social skills related to the workplace environment are uniquely under the purview of SLPs (Meulenbroek et al., 2016). Understanding the social scripts and social and cognitive demands of the workplace are important for developing treatment targets for self-schema, work-schema, as well as the placement of these factors in the person's work domain priorities. It is also essential

Workplace Job Analysis Worksheet

Importance	Frequency
0 = Not performed	0 = Not performed
1 = Not important	1 = Every few months
2 = Somewhat important	2 = Every few weeks
3 = Important	3 = Every few days (weekly)
4 = Very Important	4 = Every few hours (daily)
5 = Extremely Important	5 = Hourly

Task	Source	Importance	Frequency

Figure 8–3. A workplace job analysis can be developed to identify the importance and frequency with which communication interactions happen in the workplace. The task performance criteria should be confirmed with the client's employer, but the source of each task can be from the client, coworkers, or the supervisor (Homa & DeLambo, 2015).

to understand the workplace culture (Hagner, 2000; Homa & DeLambo, 2015; Phillips et al., 2018). Some things to consider include: (1) Are there tasks that two or more workers perform together? (2) Are there tasks that almost everyone does (sending e-mails, delivering orders to the cook, etc.)? (3) Is there a set work schedule? (4) Who evaluates whom regarding work performance and how is this rated? (5) Are there common areas and breaks that occur? (6) How do coworkers interact? These and other cultural questions about the makeup of the workplace can be used to establish its appropriateness and, hopefully, avoid difficulties due to personality mismatches.

Professional workplace communication skills are generally highly valued by employers and can be trained regardless of workplace culture (Meulenbroek & Cherney, 2019). An individual who sustains a TBI as an adolescent might not have a well-developed social schema of workplace social skills. Teaching general conversational strategies emphasizing cooperativity between conversation partners may be important and could include terminology that avoids certitude (e.g., "This is the way we do things here," versus "While you are here we suggest you go about things in this manner"). Video or audio recordings of role-play interactions that include informing others, giving feedback, receiving feedback, and clarifying miscommunications can be helpful for review with the client (Hoepner & Olson, 2018). Activities for such interactions can be found in materials for English as a second language or on human resources websites. Such role-play scenarios can be adapted for the specific issues the clinician may wish to target.

Family

Families have different configurations, different values, and different roles within them. Life after TBI typically includes changes to these relationships, roles, and responsibilities. Changes in roles may include a family member assuming power of attorney, or the person with TBI no longer being responsible for planning the family vacation. The degree to which these changes affect the person with TBI are not predictable; the person with TBI may feel that inability to plan the family vacation is more debilitating than having another family member make medical and financial decisions on their behalf.

In the *Centeredness Theory Interview* the SLP should inquire about family schemas. The SLP might probe for roles that the individual plays in their family's event planning or managing day-to-day activities. For instance, difficulties with emotional regulation or impulsivity could result in changes in child rearing. Family members might now be responsible for transportation, encouraging the person with TBI to continue with therapy or to increase their social engagement (Gagnon, Lin, & Stergiou-Kita, 2016). Challenges in communication affects an essential element for family connections. Probing for stressors that impact family members will enable the SLP to make appropriate referrals for psychological needs and identify possible targets for intervention. Creating goals focused on increasing the consistency and accuracy of family duties and responsibilities may support a client's participation within the family.

Family members might view the person with TBI as very different from whom they were before their injury (Godwin, Kreutzer, Arango-Lasprilla, & Lehan, 2011). Together with role changes, this can lead to resentment and frustration that erodes family relationships. The literature on the resilience of marriage after TBI is mixed (Godwin et al., 2011; Gosling & Oddy, 1999). Some research shows that women of partners with TBI are significantly less satisfied with relationships than their spouses with TBI (Gosling & Oddy, 1999). Other research shows that marital satisfaction levels can remain high after injury (Godwin et al., 2011). Sometimes playing the role of both caregiver and spouse, or caregiver and father, can complicate communication styles. For instance, a family member may believe that using a therapeutic approach for memory is a good way to be supportive. However, interactions that assume the form of consistent quizzing that challenge the person with TBI may become frustrating for both conversation partners.

Communication partner training directly targets the communication patterns of conversation partners. Programs such as TBI Express (Togher, McDonald, Tate, Power, & Rietdijk, 2013) and TBIconneCT (Rietdijk, Power, Brunner, & Togher, 2019) provide clinicians with interventions to train communication partners of those with TBI, in person or virtually, positively impacting the family environment. Furthermore, recent group treatment programs, such as that described by Keegan, Murdock, Suger, and Togher (2019) allow for individuals to practice communicating with peers in typical communication environments. Group interactions can support identity development after TBI (Keegan et al., 2017), and facilitate positive interactions within the family unit, as well as with others in their conversational community.

Relationship

Isolation of the individual with TBI and loneliness in the caregiver can result from mobility restrictions, disinterest, or social communication deficits (Kratz, Sander, Brickell, Lange, & Carlozzi, 2017). Apathy is a clinical impairment associated with TBI and can affect the desire to socialize. Interpersonal behaviors related to TBI such as impulsivity, social cue misperception, and poor social judgment and decision making may embarrass friends and restrict social circles after injury (Kratz et al., 2017).

When engaging in a *Centeredness Theory Interview,* the clinician can probe about relationships to prompt information about the desirability of new friendships, how to sustain existing friendships, or rekindle relationships that have been ignored. It is important to include family members or friends when working on socialization goals so that the communication partners will assist with supporting positive social engagement. In their antecedent-based behavior management approach, Feeney and Ylvisaker (1997) stress how negative and positive emotional cycles can develop after TBI. Positive Behavior Interventions and Supports (PBIS) target self-regulatory and executive functioning required for social appropriateness in schools and workplaces (Ylvisaker, Jacobs, & Feeney, 2003). Ylvisaker and Feeney (2000) suggest using a functional analysis of social behavior of the person with TBI, similar to the job analysis discussed earlier. A functional analysis might include exploring factors such as situational antecedents and consequences and observations of what specific teaching methods are preferred (e.g., prompting, shaping, fading, etc.) that can assist with generalization of new adaptive skills. The focus of a functional analysis would be made of clients' natural social environments as well as their relationships.

Romantic relationships can be severely affected after TBI due to hormonal changes, side effects of medication, fatigue, as well as social and cognitive communication deficits. The collaboration of a significant other in recovery is important for social identity reconstruction after TBI, as well as for developing new romantic relationships (Nochi, 2000). Sexual relationships are significantly impaired in approximately one-third of persons with TBI (Downing & Ponsford, 2018). Video playback is a potentially powerful tool in providing insight in both partners and persons with TBI as to what causes communication breakdowns (Hoepner & Olson, 2018). Video can be especially helpful for identifying aspects of physical behaviors as well as voice, intonation, and so forth, which can help the individual with TBI understand what others might see and observe in a courtship encounter.

Sexually offensive behavior occurs after injury in 3.5% to 9% of adults with TBI (Simpson, Blaszczynski, & Hodgkinson, 1999). There is generally poor agreement between persons with TBI and close others as to the presence of and need to remediate problematic behaviors, even years after injury. This indicates that recognition and/or acceptance of inappropriate behaviors can persist long after injury (Hicks et al., 2017). Proper channeling of romantic feelings is a strong motivator for persons with TBI and facilitation of appropriate social encounters that have the potential to lead to romantic partnerships should be considered as an appropriate focus for therapy.

Communication partners often feel a burden for directing and managing the coherence of conversation when communicating with a person with TBI. A sociolinguistic approach to social communication might be an appropriate way to approach these problems areas. For instance, persons with TBI use fewer mental state terms (i.e., words that convey emotions, thoughts and desires) and fewer linguistic markers for politeness (e.g., please, maybe, might, could), possibly indicating that they use fewer conversational moves that convey information about theory of mind (Byom & Turkstra, 2012; Meulenbroek & Cherney, 2019). The absence of these characteristic components of empathy (communicating wants, needs, acknowledging other's thoughts and feelings, etc.) might affect the perceived quality of conversation. Persons with communication deficits related to TBI are seen by conversation partners as more egocentric, less satisfying conversationalists, requiring more effort to converse with, and occasionally offensive or off-putting (Bond & Godfrey, 1997). The SLP might improve the interactional style of the person with TBI (Meulenbroek & Cherney, 2019) by targeting the increased use of linguistic units in treatment such as politeness markers. This may open up conversation to alternate opinions and support the emotional needs of the listener. By targeting increased use of mental state words and politeness markers, a clinician could promote the client's perspective taking and use of theory of mind in conversational routines.

Community

The ability to detect and respond appropriately to the thoughts and feelings of others is important for relationships and by extension community-mindedness for contemplating the impact of social decisions and social trajectory. Impaired emotion recognition and social decision-making associated with TBI can result in a range of behaviors of concern to a community more generally (Hicks et al., 2017). Because friendships are negotiated through communicative interactions (Eckert, 2000), and the success of communication can influence the success of relationships/friendships, social communication problems can result in societal disenfranchisement, as represented by the alarming prevalence of moderate to severe TBI in the homeless (22.5%) and TBI among incarcerated populations (40% to 60%) (Durand et al., 2017; Stubbs et al., 2020). Cognitive and communication limitations disenfranchise persons with TBI. This leads to reduced participation in previous life activities and reduced satisfaction with life. Unfortunately, this can potentially lead to a more pessimistic attitude toward the direction in which life is headed (Dijkers, 2004). Although this bleak picture is not necessarily true for all persons with moderate to severe TBI, the evidence indicates that these are all real factors affecting persons with TBI. These factors are arguably all interrelated and have been associated with the competence and quality of social interactions (Bond & Godfrey, 1997; Byom & Turkstra, 2017).

The final schema addressed in the *Centeredness Theory Interview* is community, where the SLP can probe how the individual with TBI views interacting with the world in a constructive and positive way. As time goes on after injury, persons with TBI typically depend more and more on family for social engagement for both arranging and accompanying them on outings. Identifying and encouraging relationships with volunteer and community social groups is an important aspect of rehabilitation. Engagement in brain injury support groups and clubhouse programming is an essential component of improving ties to the community at large. It is important for the SLP to provide information about available supports and services to persons with TBI (Fraas, Balz, & Degrauw, 2007). Groups for persons with TBI can also help support journaling strategies that facilitate coping strategies and ways of redefining identity after TBI (Fraas & Balz, 2008). Journal writing can happen privately, or as Fraas and Balz (2008) describe it, through narration to an SLP who can put the spoken words into writing and assist with the organization of language. In these writing encounters, persons with TBI can complete readings with others and then engage in discussions about the theme. An example provided by Fraas and Balz (2008) is reading *The Giving Tree* (Silverstein, 1992), talking about a gift that could be given to someone, then writing about it. These approaches can increase a sense of self-discovery and help individuals with TBI find the ability to put their emotions into words.

Persons with TBI need support for identifying information and resources about what social services are available to them. By facilitating resources through support groups run by SLPs or other professionals, persons with TBI can also gain access to information regarding community, private, and governmental benefits afforded to them (Trexler, Trexler, Malec, Klyce, & Parrott, 2010). The SLP must advocate for their client's communication rights as outlined in the National Joint Committee for the Communication Needs of Persons with Severe Disabilities (Brady et al., 2016). It is important that SLPs ensure that the person with TBI has access to community resources and that their communication partners are included in the rehabilitation process. This is beneficial for both the recovery of the person with the communication impairment as well as that person's larger community. Communication partner training similar to the content in TBI Express has also been explored for paid caregivers (Behn, Togher, Power, & Heard, 2012). SLPs and others can provide supported communication training for service personnel in community settings, where the person with TBI might find themselves, including hospitals, community centers, or YMCAs and local gyms.

Finally, motivation for participation in treatment and progress toward goals can often be influenced by the individual's relationship with their clinician. Clinicians need to support the client's autonomous role in identity negotiation, provide resources for successful communication of their identity, and acknowledge the role of communication partners in the communication environment, as a component of this positive identity construction. Because identity is socially constructed, it is especially relevant to the SLP, who may be one of the few communication partners who can intentionally support the individual with TBI as they strive to communicate their changing identity. The SLP has a role in creating opportunities for the individual to express who they are and assist them in describing their personal priorities, roles, and goals, in a variety of contexts. Furthermore, the SLP can put supports in place, so that individuals with TBI can work toward these individual roles and goals. Working on the development of social communication and pragmatic skills can provide an individual with a voice and an avenue through which to express their identity. Finally, although clinicians ideally strive to maintain cooperative and collaborative relationships with their clients, there remains a socially imposed power differential between the individual with a TBI seeking support, and the expert imparting aid. Thus, it is important for clinicians to remain cognizant of their influence. The SLP should refrain from imposing identities that, for the client, are not positive, and avoid emphasizing the disability so much that the client solely thinks of themselves as "impaired."

Conclusion

There is no shortcut to following best clinical practice. Client-centered practice requires an in-depth probing into the nature of current client interactions as well as future/desired interactions. Figure 8–4 depicts the types of probes that can be used

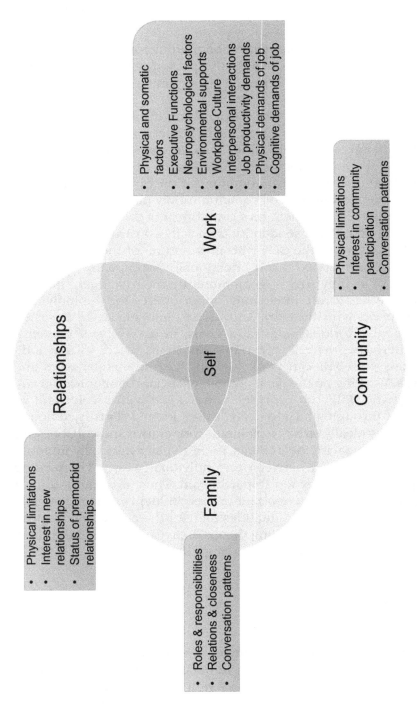

Figure 8–4. The Centeredness Theory Interview covers various aspects of an individual's social domain.

in a *Centeredness Theory Interview* that have been discussed throughout this chapter. Client-centered goal formation starts with assessment and actively listening to the client without judgment. Treatment of social and communication goals requires understanding the client's environmental and contextual supports and barriers and the potential environmental modifications that may assist the client in achieving specified goals. These principles are supported by the literature on clinical practice (Togher et al., 2014) and imply a shift from workbook-based or "cookie-cutter" treatments. The LPAA philosophy emphasizes the focus on the person, their environment, and successful participation in life from the perspective of the client. Living successfully with communication impairment means communicating in a manner that is acceptable to the individual with TBI. In a paradox that must be embraced, independence after TBI relies heavily on the support of others in the individual's family, social circles, workplace, and community.

References

Adolphs, R. (2009). The social brain: Neural basis of social knowledge. *Annual Review of Psychology, 60*, 693–716. https://doi.org/10.1146/annurev.psych.60.110707.163514

Allain, P., Togher, L., & Azouvi, P. (2018). Social cognition and traumatic brain injury: Current knowledge. *Brain Injury, 33*(1), 1–3. https://doi.org/10.1080/02699052.2018.1533143

Beaulieu-Bonneau, S., & Morin, C. M. (2012). Sleepiness and fatigue following traumatic brain injury. *Sleep Medicine, 13*(6), 598–605. https://doi.org/10.1016/j.sleep.2012.02.010

Behn, N., Togher, L., Power, E., & Heard, R. (2012). Evaluating communication training for paid careers of people with traumatic brain injury. *Brain Injury, 26*(13-14), 1702–1715. https://doi.org/10.3109/02699052.2012.722258

Bloch-Jorgensen, Z. T., Cilione, P. J., Yeung, W. W. H., & Gatt, J. M. (2018). Centeredness Theory: Understanding and measuring well-being across core life domains. *Frontiers in Psychology, 9*, 610. https://doi.org/10.3389/fpsyg.2018.00610

Bond, F., & Godfrey, H. P. D. (1997). Conversation with traumatically brain-injured individuals: A controlled study of behavioural changes and their impact. *Brain Injury, 11*(5), 319–329. https://doi.org/10.1080/026990597123476

Brady, N. C., Bruce, S., Goldman, A., Erickson, K., Mineo, B., Ogletree, B. T., . . . Wilkinson, K. (2016). Communication services and supports for individuals with severe disabilities: Guidance for assessment and intervention. *American Journal on Intellectual and Developmental Disability, 121*(2), 121–138. https://doi.org/10.1352/1944-7558-121.2.121

Byom, L. J., O'Neil-Pirozzi, T., Lemoncello, R., MacDonald, S., Meulenbroek, P., Ness, B., & Sohlberg, M. M. (in press). Social communication following adult traumatic brain injury: A scoping review of theoretical models. *American Journal of Speech-Language Pathology.*

Byom, L. J., & Turkstra, L. S. (2012). Effects of social cognitive demand on Theory of Mind in conversations of adults with traumatic brain injury. *International Journal of Language & Communication Disorders, 47*(3), 310–321.

Byom, L. J., & Turkstra, L. S. (2017). Cognitive task demands and discourse performance after traumatic brain injury. *International Journal of Language & Communication Disorders, 52*(4), 501–513. https://doi.org/10.1111/1460-6984.12289

Constantinidou, F., Wertheimer, J. C., Tsanadis, J., Evans, C., & Paul, D. R. (2012). Assessment of executive functioning in brain injury: Collaboration between speech-language pathology and neuropsychology for an integrative neuropsychological perspective. *Brain Injury, 26*(13-14), 1549–1563. https://doi.org/10.3109/02699052.2012.698786

Crosson, B., Barco, P. P., Velozo, C. A., Bolesta, M. M., Cooper, P. V., Werts, D., & Brokbeck, T. C. (1989). Awareness and compensation in postacute head injury rehabilitation. *The Journal Head Trauma Rehabilitation, 4*(3), 46–54.

Dean, P. J., & Sterr, A. (2013). Long-term effects of mild traumatic brain injury on cognitive performance. *Frontiers in Human Neuroscience, 7*, 30. https://doi.org/10.3389/fnhum.2013.00030

Diener, E., Wirtz, D., Tov, W., Kim-Prieto, C., Choi, D.-w., Oishi, S., & Biswas-Diener, R. (2010). New well-being measures: Short scales to assess flourishing and positive and negative feelings. *Social Indicators Research, 97*(2), 143–156. http:// doi:10.1007/s11205-009-9493-y

Dijkers, M. P. (2004). Quality of life after traumatic brain injury: A review of research approaches and findings. *Archives of Physical Medicine and Rehabilitation, 85*(Suppl. 2), 21–35.

Dikmen, S. S., Temkin, N. R., Machamer, J. E., & Holubkov, A. L. (1994). Employment following traumatic head injuries. *Archives of Neurology, 51*(2), 177–186.

Downing, M., & Ponsford, J. (2018). Sexuality in individuals with traumatic brain injury and their partners. *Neuropsychological Rehabilitation*, *28*(6), 1028–1037. https://doi.org/10.1080/09602011.2016.123 6732

Durand, E., Chevignard, M., Ruet, A., Dereix, A., Jourdan, C., & Pradat-Diehl, P. (2017). History of traumatic brain injury in prison populations: A systematic review. *Annals of Physical and Rehabilitation Medicine*, *60*(2), 95–101. https://doi.org/10.1016/j.rehab.2017.02.003

Eckert, P. (2000). *Linguistic variation as social practice*. Malden, MA: Blackwell.

Feeney, T. J., & Ylvisaker, M. (1997). A positive, communication-based approach to challenging behavior after ABI. In A. Glang, G. H. S. Singer, & B. Todis (Eds.), *Students with acquired brain injury: The school's response* (pp. 229–254). Baltimore, MD: Brookes.

Fraas, M., & Balz, M. A. (2008). Expressive electronic journal writing: Freedom of communication for survivors of acquired brain injury. *Journal of Psycholinguistic Research*, *37*(2), 115–124. https://doi .org/10.1007/s10936-007-9062-y

Fraas, M., Balz, M., & Degrauw, W. (2007). Meeting the long-term needs of adults with acquired brain injury through community-based programming. *Brain Injury*, *21*(12), 1267–1281. https://doi.org/10 .1080/02699050701721794

Gagnon, A., Lin, J., & Stergiou-Kita, M. (2016). Family members facilitating community re-integration and return to productivity following traumatic brain injury—motivations, roles and challenges. *Disability and Rehabilitation*, *38*(5), 433–441. https://doi.org/10.3109/09638 288.2015.1044035

Godwin, E. E., Kreutzer, J. S., Arango-Lasprilla, J. C., & Lehan, T. J. (2011). Marriage after brain injury: Review, analysis, and research recommendations. *The Journal of Head Trauma Rehabilitation*, *26*(1), 43–55. https://doi.org/10.1097/HTR.0b013e3182048f54

Gosling, J., & Oddy, M. (1999). Rearranged marriages: Marital relationships after head injury. *Brain Injury*, *13*(10), 785–796.

Gray, J. M., Shepherd, M., McKinlay, W. W., Robertson, I., & Pentland, B. (1994). Negative symptoms in the traumatically brain-injured during the first year postdischarge, and their effect on rehabilitation status, work status and family burden. *Clinical Rehabilitation*, *8*(3), 188–197.

Hagner, D. (2000). *Coffee breaks and birthday cakes: Evaluating workplace cultures to develop natural supports for employees with disabilities*. St. Augustine, FL: Training Resource Network.

Hart, T., Ketchum, J. M., O'Neil-Pirozzi, T. M., Novack, T. A., Johnson-Greene, D., & Dams-O'Connor, K. (2019). Neurocognitive status and return to work after moderate to severe traumatic brain injury. *Rehabilitation Psychology, 64*(4), 435–444. https://doi.org/ 10.1037/ rep0000290

Hicks, A. J., Gould, K. R., Hopwood, M., Kenardy, J., Krivonos, I., & Ponsford, J. L. (2017). Behaviours of concern following moderate to severe traumatic brain injury in individuals living in the community. *Brain Injury*, 1–8. https://doi.org/10.1080/02699052.2017.1317361

Hoepner, J. K., & Olson, S. E. (2018). Joint video self-modeling as a conversational intervention for an Individual with traumatic brain injury and his everyday partner: A pilot investigation. *Clinical Archives of Communication Disorders, 3*(1), 22–41. https://doi.org/10.21849/ cacd.2018.00262

Homa, D., & DeLambo, D. (2015). Vocational assessment and job placement. In R. Escorpizo, S. Brage, D. Homa, & G. Stucki (Eds.), *Handbook of vocational rehabilitation and disability evaluation: Application and implementation of the ICF* (pp. 161–186). Cham, Switzerland: Springer International.

Kagan, A., & Simmons-Mackie, N. (2007). Beginning with the end: Outcome-driven assessment and intervention with life participation in mind. *Topics in Language Disorders, 27*(4), 309–317.

Kagan, A., Simmons-Mackie, N., Rowland, A., Huijbregts, M., Shumway, E., McEwen, S., . . . Sharp, S. (2008). Counting what counts: A framework for capturing real-life outcomes of aphasia intervention. *Aphasiology, 22*(3), 258–280.

Keegan, L. C., Murdock, M., Suger, C., & Togher, L. (2019). Improving natural social interaction: Group rehabilitation after traumatic brain injury. *Neuropsychological Rehabilitation*, 1–26. https://doi.org/10 .1080/09602011.2019.1591464

Keegan, L. C., Togher, L., Murdock, M., & Hendry, E. (2017). Expression of masculine identity in individuals with a traumatic brain injury. *Brain Injury, 31*(12), 1632–1641. https://doi.org/10.1080/02699052 .2017.1332389

Kennedy, M. (2017). *Coaching college students with executive function problems*. New York, NY: Guilford Press.

Kennedy, M. R., & Coelho, C. (2005). Self-regulation after traumatic brain injury: A framework for intervention of memory and problem solving. *Seminars in Speech and Language, 26*(4), 242–255. https:// doi.org/10.1055/s-2005-922103

Kratz, A. L., Sander, A. M., Brickell, T. A., Lange, R. T., & Carlozzi, N. E. (2017). Traumatic brain injury caregivers: A qualitative analysis of spouse and parent perspectives on quality of life. *Neuropsychological Rehabilitation, 27*(1), 16–37. https://doi.org/10.1080/09602011 .2015.1051056

LPAA Project Group (Chapey, R., Duchan, J., Elman, R., Garcia, L., Kagan, A., Lyon, J., & Simmons-Mackie, N.). (2000). Life participation approach to aphasia: A statement of values. *ASHA Leader, 5*(3), 4–6. https://doi.org/10.1044/leader.FTR.05032000.4

Lundahl, B., Droubay, B. A., Burke, B., Butters, R. P., Nelford, K., Hardy, C., . . . Bowles, M. (2019). Motivational interviewing adherence tools: A scoping review investigating content validity. *Patient Education and Counseling, 102*(12), 2145–2155. https://doi.org/10.1016/j.pec.2019.07.003

MacQueen, R., Fisher, P., & Williams, D. (2018). A qualitative investigation of masculine identity after traumatic brain injury. *Neuropsychological Rehabilitation*, 1–17. https://doi.org/10.1080/09602011.2018.1466714

McAllister, T. W. (1992). Neuropsychiatric sequelae of head injuries. *The Psychiatric Clinics of North America, 15*(2), 395–413.

McDonald, S., Honan, C., Kelly, M., Byom, L. J., & Rushby, J. (2014). Disorders of social cognition and social behaviour following severe TBI. In S. McDonald, L. Togher, & C. Code (Eds.), *Social and communication disorders following traumatic brain injury* (2nd ed., pp. 119–159). London, UK: Psychology Press.

Meulenbroek, P., Bowers, B., & Turkstra, L. S. (2016). Characterizing common workplace communication skills for disorders associated with traumatic brain injury: A qualitative study. *Journal of Vocational Rehabilitation, 44*(1), 15–31. https://doi.org/10.3233/JVR-150777

Meulenbroek, P., & Cherney, L. R. (2019). The voicemail elicitation task: Functional workplace language assessment for persons with traumatic brain injury. *Journal of Speech, Language, and Hearing Research, 62*(9), 1–14. https://doi.org/10.1044/2019_jslhr-l-18-0466

Meulenbroek, P., Ness, B., Lemoncello, R., Byom, L., MacDonald, S., O'Neil-Pirozzi, T. M., & Sohlberg, M. M. (2019). Social communication following traumatic brain injury, part 2: Identifying effective social communication treatment ingredients. *International Journal Speech-Language Pathology, 21*(2), 128–142. https://doi.org/10.1080/17549507.2019.1583281

Meulenbroek, P., & Turkstra, L. S. (2016). Job stability in skilled work and communication ability after moderate-severe traumatic brain injury. *Disability Rehabilitation, 38*(5), 452–461. https://doi.org/10.3109/09638288.2015.1044621

Miller, W. R., & Rollnick, S. (2013). *Motivational interviewing: Helping people change* (3rd ed.). New York, NY: Guilford Press.

Nochi, M. (2000). Reconstructing self-narratives in coping with traumatic brain injury. *Social Science & Medicine, 51*(12), 1795–1804.

Ownsworth, T. (2014). *Self-identity after brain injury.* New York, NY: Taylor & Francis Group.

Phillips, B. N., Reyes, A., Kriofske Mainella, A. M., Kesselmayer, R. F., & Jacobson, J. D. (2018). A needs driven model of workplace social effectiveness in adults with disabilities. *Rehabilitation Counseling Bulletin, 62*(1), 30–42. https://doi.org/10.1177/0034355217747690.

Prien, E. P., Goodstein, L. D., Goodstein, J., & Gamble, L. G. (2009). *A practical guide to job analysis.* San Francisco, CA: Pfeiffer.

Rietdijk, R., Power, E., Brunner, M., & Togher, L. (2019). A single case experimental design study on improving social communication skills after traumatic brain injury using communication partner telehealth training. *Brain Injury, 33*(1), 94–104. https://doi.org/10.1080/0269 9052.2018.1531313

Silverstein, S. (1992). *The giving tree.* New York, NY: HarperCollins.

Simpson, G., Blaszczynski, A., & Hodgkinson, A. (1999). Sex offending as a psychosocial sequela of traumatic brain injury. *The Journal of Head Trauma Rehabilitation, 14*(6), 567–580. https://doi.org/ 10.1097/00001199-199912000-00005

Stubbs, J. L., Thornton, A. E., Sevick, J. M., Silverberg, N. D., Barr, A. M., Honer, W. G., & Panenka, W. J. (2020). Traumatic brain injury in homeless and marginally housed individuals: A systematic review and meta-analysis. *Lancet Public Health, 5*(1), e19–e32. https://doi .org/10.1016/s2468-2667(19)30188-4

Togher, L., Hand, L., & Code, C. (1996). A new perspective on the relationship between communication impairment and disempowerment following head injury in information exchanges. *Disability and Rehabilitation, 18*(11), 559–566.

Togher, L., McDonald, S., Tate, R., Power, E., & Rietdijk, R. (2013). Training communication partners of people with severe traumatic brain injury improves everyday conversations: A multicenter single blind clinical trial. *Journal of Rehabilitation Medicine.* https://doi .org/10.2340/16501977-1173

Togher, L., Wiseman-Hakes, C., Douglas, J., Stergiou-Kita, M., Ponsford, J., Teasell, R., . . . Turkstra, L. S. (2014). INCOG recommendations for management of cognition following traumatic brain injury, part IV: Cognitive communication. *The Journal of Head Trauma Rehabilitation, 29*(4), 353–368. https://doi.org/10.1097/htr.0000000000000071

Trexler, L. E., Trexler, L. C., Malec, J. F., Klyce, D., & Parrott, D. (2010). Prospective randomized controlled trial of resource facilitation on community participation and vocational outcome following brain injury. *The Journal of Head Trauma Rehabilitation, 25*(6), 440–446. https://doi.org/10.1097/HTR.0b013e3181d41139

Turkstra, L. S. (2008). Conversation-based assessment of social cognition in adults with traumatic brain injury. *Brain Injury, 22*(5), 397–409.

Turkstra, L. S., Clark, A., Burgess, S., Hengst, J. A., Wertheimer, J. C., & Paul, D. (2017). Pragmatic communication abilities in children and adults: Implications for rehabilitation professionals. *Disability and Rehabilitation, 39*(18), 1872–1885. https://doi.org/10.1080/09638288 .2016.1212113

Turkstra, L. S., McDonald, S., & DePompei, R. (2001). Social information processing in adolescents: Data from normally developing adolescents and preliminary data from their peers with traumatic brain injury. *Journal of Head Trauma Rehabilitation, 16*(5), 469–483.

Turkstra, L. S., Norman, R., Whyte, J., Dijkers, M. P., & Hart, T. (2016). Knowing what we're doing: Why specification of treatment methods is critical for evidence-based practice in speech-language pathology. *American Journal of Speech-Language Pathology, 25*(2), 164–171. https://doi.org/10.1044/2015_ajslp-15-0060

Turner-Stokes, L., Williams, H., & Johnson, J. (2009). Goal attainment scaling: Does it provide added value as a person-centred measure for evaluation of outcome in neurorehabilitation following acquired brain injury? *Journal of Rehabilitation Medicine, 41*(7), 528–535. https://doi.org/10.2340/16501977-0383

Worthington, A., & Wood, R. L. (2018). Apathy following traumatic brain injury: A review. *Neuropsychologia, 118*(Pt. B), 40–47. https://doi .org/10.1016/j.neuropsychologia.2018.04.012

Ylvisaker, M. (2006). Self-coaching: A context-sensitive, person-centred *(sic)* approach to social communication after traumatic brain injury. *Brain Impairment, 7*(3), 246–258. https://doi.org/10.1375/brim.7 .3.246

Ylvisaker, M., & Feeney, T. (2000). Reconstruction of identity after brain injury. *Brain Impairment, 1*(1), 12–28.

Ylvisaker, M., Feeney, T. J., & Urbanczyk, B. (1993). Developing a positive communication culture for rehabilitation: Communication training for staff and family members. In C. J. Durgin, N. D. Schmidt, & L. J. Fryer (Eds.), *Staff development and clinical intervention in brain injury rehabilitation.* (pp. 57–85). Gaithersburg, MD: Aspen.

Ylvisaker, M., Jacobs, H. E., & Feeney, T. (2003). Positive supports for people who experience behavioral and cognitive disability after brain injury: A review. *The Journal of Head Trauma Rehabilitation, 18*(1), 7–32. https://doi.org/10.1097/00001199-200301000-00005

Young, J. E. (1994). *Cognitive therapy for personality disorders: A schema-focused approach* (Rev. ed.). Sarasota, FL: Professional Resource Press.

9

THE LIFE PARTICIPATION APPROACH TO APHASIA

LOOKING BACK AND MOVING FORWARD

Nina Simmons-Mackie

The Life Participation Approach to Aphasia (LPAA) is officially 20 years old (see Prologue for reprint of LPAA Project Group, 2000). But, as described in the introductory chapters, the evolution toward LPAA began much earlier with attention to functional communication, pragmatics, and social theory, as well as recognition by clinicians of the pressing need to improve how people with aphasia experience their lives and reintegrate into the community. This movement toward making sure people are living life to their potential is the crux of the Social Imperative.

I originally became deeply interested in the Social Imperative after analyzing aphasia therapy interactions using qualitative research methods (e.g., Simmons-Mackie & Damico, 1993, 1999, 2011; Simmons-Mackie, Damico, & Nelson, 1995). What I discovered was a very "therapist-centered" approach in which therapists chose goals, materials, activities, and the time allotted to tasks. Therapists initiated talk and directed the flow of interaction. I wondered "how are people with aphasia supposed to learn how to manage their own communication when interaction is controlled by the speech-language pathologist (SLP)"? Fortunately, motivated and thoughtful clinicians and researchers have effected many changes in practices over the last decades. In fact, a seismic change has occurred in health care philosophy generally, with wide philosophical acceptance of patient-centered health care.

LPAA is consistent with this patient-centered health care movement (I will use the label "person-centered care" (PCC) henceforth). Recall that LPAA is a "consumer driven" set of values that places the needs and wants of people living with aphasia at the forefront. As LPAA and the person-centered philosophy advanced, it became accepted that clinicians should appreciate and understand people with aphasia as living in the context of their own social worlds; as people who must be listened to, informed, respected; and as people who should be meaningfully involved in their own therapy (Epstein & Street, 2011, p. 100). LPAA also involves family and friends, considers cultural context, and focuses on an environment that supports participation and well-being. In other words, LPAA is a holistic approach to intervention that is based on specific values and principles that fulfill the call of the Social Imperative. Although LPAA values were proposed for aphasia, these values are widely relevant. Hence the attention in this book centers on aphasia (including primary progressive aphasia), traumatic brain injury (TBI) and dementia. I will focus largely on aphasia, but most of my thoughts are more widely applicable.

Has LPAA impacted clinical practice? Where are we headed? Looking forward to the next 20 years, there are obvious, and perhaps less obvious themes, and good news, as well as worries. This chapter will outline some of the opportunities to advance the Social Imperative and LPAA. Many of these opportunities are reflected in themes that reverberate through this book such as attention to choices, meaningful activities, the environment, care partners, and emotional health.

Choice

An emphasis on choice is both an explicit and implicit theme in this book. Choice, or the freedom to be oneself and do what one chooses, is closely tied to one's identity, self-confidence, and well-being. Choices reflect who we are and what we value. The Social Imperative weaves client choice throughout rehabilitation. For example, Douglas and Smyth (Chapter 7; 2021) advise that an evidence-based approach in dementia care involves clients "choosing activities based on their preferences" and engaging "blocks of activity time based upon their own desires, not the desires of an institution or family member." Similarly, Sather and Howe (Chapter 4; 2021) suggest that "voluntariness" (i.e., opportunity to make choices) is an important attribute of a rich and stimulating environment that enhances well-being for people with aphasia.

One of the most critical issues of choice faced in intervention is choice of goal(s). An appropriate process of goal setting within PCC and LPAA is a collaboration between the SLP and the client. In the past, it has been reported that goals were chosen by clinicians, that clients were rarely aware of their goals, and that goals were often distant from daily needs (e.g., Parr, Byng, Gilpin, & Ireland, 1997; Simmons-Mackie & Damico, 1999). People with aphasia reported that the direction of therapy was often confusing, or the content seemed irrelevant (Hersh, 2004; Parr et al., 1997). I recall Susie Parr describing a person's response to her query about what he had gotten out of aphasia therapy; he stated "I never knew what a verb was. Now I do!"

Although we have made progress in clinician attitude and beliefs about PCC and shared decision making (e.g., Rose, Ferguson, Power, Togher, & Worrall, 2014), collaborative goal setting remains elusive in daily practice (e.g., Rohde, Townley-O'Neill, Trendall, Worrall, & Cornwell, 2012). SLPs and other rehabilitation clinicians continue to report difficulty with collaborative goal setting (Berg, Askim, Balandin, Armstrong, & Rise, 2017; Berg, Rise, Balandin, Armstrong, & Askim, 2016; Holliday, Antoun, & Playford, 2005). Goal setting "collaborations" are often superficial, not only in aphasia therapy, but in health care in general. For example, although client signatures on written goal statements may be taken as evidence of the client "participating" in goal setting, the fact is that the goals were created by the clinician and simply acquiesced to by the client (The Joint Commission, 2016).

Suggestions for how to manage true client collaboration are emerging. In this book, authors make suggestions for setting goals that reflect the real-life preferences and choices of the client with aphasia. Elman (Chapter 2; 2021) describes C.A.P.E.—one potential guide for goal setting discussions. Baar (Chapter 3; 2021) and Meulenbroek and Keegan (Chapter 8; 2021) suggest using "motivational interviewing." Strong and Shadden (Chapter 5; 2021) encourage clinicians to listen to and support people with aphasia in telling stories that provide personally meaningful direction for intervention. Sather and Howe (Chapter 4; 2021) reference the collaborative FOURC model of goal setting (Haley, Cunningham, Barry, & de Riesthal. 2019), the use of semi-structured interviews with conversational supports, or the *Assessment for Living with Aphasia* (Kagan et al., 2011) to identify meaningful participation goals.

We are moving forward! There has clearly been progress in considering that each person brings to treatment their unique perspectives and wishes that must be integrated into goals. Researchers and program developers are beginning to recognize the need to meaningfully include people living with aphasia as coparticipants in the design of programs and the choice of programming solutions (Konnerup, 2017; McMenamin, Tierney, & MacFarlane, 2018; Pound & Laywood, 2020). The voices of people living with aphasia are beginning to emerge. Changes in SLP conceptions of goal setting are emerging. For example, Haley and colleagues (2019), give examples of client goals such: as "show my intelligence,"; "talk as if I don't have aphasia at my class reunion"; "respond to text messages by myself." These are personally meaningful goals! With the identification of such goals, therapy could take many directions, and the achievement of a specific goal would likely impact other activities through improvements in language, confidence, and strategy use.

But, let's imagine what can be accomplished in the next 20 years. Collaboration with people with marked communication disability is challenging, and clients might feel unprepared to make choices about their treatment. We will need to create practical resources and guides of exactly how collaboration is accomplished. Significant change will need to occur in the training of clinicians and students. Explicit techniques and resources for engaging people with aphasia in goal setting and clinical decisions must be incorporated into coursework. Student training must provide *actual experiences* in implementation of PCC and shared decision making. For example, the use of "standardized patients" or virtual experiences might help promote learning of person-centered interactions (Epstein & Street, 2011; Srinivasan et al., 2006). Clinicians will need to embrace an

> expanded role in goal setting and therapy interactions . . . one where the client's voice is not only heard through the process but shapes it. Rehabilitation would be more of an enduring partnership responsive to the changing needs of an evolving disability experience" (Hersh, Sherratt et al., 2012, p. 983).

Therefore, my vision for the next 20 years would be for all clinicians and researchers to successfully and meaningfully engage clients in the goal setting, planning, and therapeutic process—not only to provide choices, but also to empower those living with aphasia to take charge of their futures.

Meaningful Outcomes

Closely related to "choice" and goal setting, is the importance of meaningful outcomes. Therefore, not surprisingly, a resounding theme in this volume is the critical importance of working toward personally meaningful outcomes. The theme is consistent across chapters, but the particulars of implementing a participation-oriented approach vary across disorders. For example, language supports are most appropriate for aphasia, whereas memory supports help people with dementia and TBI. But the general idea is to reach outside of our clinical zone of comfort (beyond the language impairment) to understand a person's context and individual daily lives and consider what approach will make a difference *there*.

Focusing on meaningful outcomes is critical to the quality of our services. In fact, throughout health care, quality of services is being redefined based on quality outcomes; a "good outcome is defined in terms of what is meaningful and valuable to the individual patient" (Epstein & Street, 2011, p. 100; Guyatt, Montori, Devereaux, Schünemann, & Bhandari, 2004). Additionally, meaningful must be defined in terms of the impact on one's daily life. Improvement in naming common objects is meaningful *only* if that person has also improved in using those words to have a conversation, negotiate a purchase, make a shopping list, or perform other activities of personal value. Meaningful outcomes also include negotiating social relationships. Communicating with family and friends is imperative for well-being; in fact, social isolation is associated with a constellation of negative health consequences (Simmons-Mackie, 2018). Integrating social connections and activities of choice into intervention goals is one key to ensuring meaningful outcomes.

How are we doing in addressing personally meaningful outcomes for people with aphasia? The good news is that clinicians generally agree that intervention should have a positive impact on functional communication and life participation; clinicians want to incorporate participation into their clinical practice (Berg et al., 2016; Hersh et al., 2012). The bad news is that participation goals are rarely targets of aphasia intervention (Simmons-Mackie, 2018; Torrence, Baylor, Yorkston, & Spencer, 2016). Clinicians have expressed frustration with the inability to work at the level of participation for a variety of reasons (Berg et al., 2016; Rose et al., 2014). Baar (Chapter 3; 2021) notes common barriers to participation-oriented intervention such as the misconception that it is not relevant until later stages of recovery; she provides a variety of practical suggestions for adjusting practice. Another common misconception is that LPAA involves *only* direct work on participation in meaningful activities. LPAA involves working on explicitly defined participation *goals* via whatever means will make a difference. For example, instead of generic words such as woman or dog, naming therapy might target personally relevant words such as family and pet names, preferred food or beverage items (Chardonnay, French fries), or favorite places (Walmart, Home Depot) (Sutton, 2020). Naming therapy might accompany work on functional phrases and use of graphic or technology supports that aim towards participating in a favored activity or role. Conversation therapy might incorporate targeted word finding or other linguistic goals. Advanced technology will help people with communication disability navigate the Internet, craft and understand e-mails, and communicate with others face-to-face. Applications of mobile technology and online resources are being described (Baier, Hoepner, & Sather, 2018; King, 2013; Szabo & Dittelman, 2014); as people become more comfortable with this technology in general, applications in communication disability will expand.

But creative intervention aimed at participation goals is not the only target for future development. Clinicians must be able to document achievement of such outcomes for funding and accountability. Suggestions for documenting outcomes are offered in several chapters, including interviewing, goal attainment scaling, using Life Interests and Values cards (Haley, Womack, Helm-Estabrooks, Lovette, & Goff, 2013), or participation measures such as the *Assessment for Living with Aphasia* (Kagan et al., 2011). Funders (and clinicians) must learn that participation outcomes ARE medically necessary because they impact health and well-being, help prevent depression, and likely reduce long-term health care costs. In the next 20 years, funders must be educated to accept person-specific goal achievement and patient report as valid, and in fact, essential for attaining personally meaningful outcomes. Clinicians will increasingly use these approaches to fulfill quality initiatives. The surging field of technology will help us track real life outcomes through wearable cameras, microphones, digital data gathering, and automated motivational devices, such as a version of Fitbit, for conversational practice (e.g., Brandenburg, Worrall, Copland, & Rodriguez, 2017).

The Environment

In addition to individual and group treatment that focuses on meaningful participation goals, the importance of the environment *around* the person with aphasia is a significant theme of the Social Imperative. The environment includes the physical and social factors in the home and the community at large. It also involves the critical role of the *opportunity* for participation that is not only enjoyable, but also healing (Armour, Brady, Sayyad, & Krieger, 2019). Aphasia camps as described by Sather & Howe (Chapter 4; 2021) are increasingly offering intervention, social connections, education, and fun for people with aphasia and their partners (e.g., Kim, Ruelling, Garcia, & Kainer, 2017). A growing number of aphasia community centers are appearing with offerings across the activity spectrum providing opportunities for supported conversation, engagement in hobbies (e.g., painting, theater, music), and social connections. Other flourishing opportunities for participation include "aphasia choirs" and supported "book clubs" (e.g., Bernstein-Ellis & Elman, 2006; Knollman-Porter & Julien, 2019; Tamplin, Baker, Jones, Way, & Lee, 2013; Zumbansen et al., 2017).

In the past 20 years, we have made significant strides in attention to the communication environment. But we have a way to go. The effort to make health care communicatively accessible is visible in the literature, but rarely visible in health care settings. Communicative access for people with aphasia (or other communication disabilities) in the wider community remains poor. My vision for the future would be an explosion of supportive environments that provide positive experiences and enhance well-being and social connections. In addition, I hope for increased success in building public awareness of aphasia and ensuring that people with aphasia have full access to life and positive experiences as they navigate public spaces and community activities. Wouldn't it be wonderful if someone with aphasia, dementia, or TBI could enter a pharmacy, a doctor's office, or department store and find people who are not only accepting, but also knowledgeable about facilitating communication and foster empowering interactions?

Care Partners

Another theme that permeates this book is the critical importance of involving care partners (i.e., family members, caretakers) in the therapy process. People are an aspect of the environment around the person with aphasia. Chapters in this book tout the importance of training partners to support communication with people with aphasia, dementia, and TBI. However, a research-to-practice gap continues in the implementation of Communication Partner Training (CPT) in clinical practice. In a survey of practices, SLPs reported low levels of CPT use and poor confidence in delivering CPT (Rose et al., 2014). Researchers have found that a lack of skills and resources were barriers to providing evidence-based CPT programs (Chang, Power, O'Halloran, & Foster, 2018). Since clinicians are *ethically bound* to ensure that care partners know how to support communication (Simmons-Mackie, 2013), we must find ways to bridge the research to practice gap. However, CPT is not only infrequent in daily clinical practices, but also clinical SLPs are often unskilled in supporting the communication of their clients. At a recent conference, I witnessed several SLPs present to an audience of people with aphasia and their families in a "nonaphasia friendly" manner using rapid rate, professional jargon, and slides crowded with text. How can we expect families to communicate successfully with their loved ones, when we aren't modeling effective supported communication? My wish for the future is that all clinicians will demonstrate skill in supporting conversation and that CPT will become a fundamental feature of SLP services. It is likely that these services will be delivered face-to-face, as well as through novel methods such as interactive on-line learning, avatar delivered training, or mixed/virtual reality experiences.

But supporting communication is not the only issue for families of people with communication disabilities. Attention to care partners is important for the well-being of the care partner as well as the well-being of the person with aphasia, dementia, or TBI. We have heard for decades that aphasia is a family disorder (as are TBI and dementia). Family members not only experience changes in lifestyle and roles, but also often experience social isolation, exhaustion, illness, and depression (Simmons-Mackie, 2018). Grawburg and colleagues (2013, 2014) describe these negative changes in functioning of the family member as "third-party disability." In fact, if those around the person are not sufficiently knowledgeable, healthy, and supported, then outcomes of the person with the communication disability will be less desirable. Yet clinicians rarely have explicit goals for family members (Sherratt et al., 2011), and family members are not typically considered a focal point of rehabilitation (Halle, LeDorze, & Mingant, 2014). Family members report feeling marginalized and unsupported (Halle et al., 2014; Howe et al., 2012; Paul & Sanders, 2010; Sherratt et al., 2011). This is likely due to lack of clinician time, resources, or funding to attend to the needs of care partners. In a white paper addressing gaps in services and recommendations for the future, improving services for family and caregivers was one of the top ten recommendations (Simmons-Mackie, 2018).

In the next decades, the focal point of rehabilitation will increasingly address care partner needs. We will need to identify mechanisms for meeting care partner needs in areas such as communication partner training, information, hope for the future, strategies to cope with new roles, and respite. Interprofessional practices, partnerships with counselors and social workers, and existing community services might offer potential solutions. Online resources and social networking (e.g., https://www.aphasiarecoveryconnection.net/) will be increasingly important sources for information, guidance, and social support for families (as well as people with aphasia). In addition, Strong and Shadden (Chapter 5; 2021) urge clinicians to *listen to* the stories that families tell—stories that help them gain insight and deal with life changes. SLPs tend to focus on the person with communication disability and give information to family members; but learning to listen to everyone involved can be a powerful tool to promote wellness. My dream for the next 20 years includes care partners as featured recipients of services.

Identity and Emotional Experience

The last theme that pervades discussions of the Social Imperative relates to internal factors such as identity, self-esteem, and feelings. Twenty years ago, "issues related to . . . psychosocial well-being . . . were relegated to a grey area on the fringe of aphasia management" (Simmons-Mackie, 1998, p. 233). Clinicians were recognizing the importance of psychosocial factors in communication recovery; however, there was little information about what to do about depression, anxiety, or low confidence. Progress has been made in recognition of the role of the SLP in identity and psychosocial health (Rose et al., 2014). For example, guidelines are emerging to assist clinicians in identifying and managing depression in people with aphasia (e.g., Baker et al., 2018; Kneebone, 2016). In the literature, we are seeing a shift toward preventing depression by addressing the themes discussed earlier, such as choice, care partners, environment, and meaningful participation (e.g., Worrall, 2019; Worrall et al., 2016). When people with aphasia are socially engaged and positive about the future, the potential onset of depression is reduced.

I anticipate a growing recognition of the serious impact of emotional health on communication and participation in the coming years. Clinicians will not only become more skilled at identifying mood and confidence issues, but will also become more skilled in counseling and more knowledgeable regarding management of mood and emotional issues. The beneficiaries of such expanded knowledge and practice will be those living with aphasia.

Concluding Thoughts

Since patient-centered care is one of the six key elements of quality health care defined by the Institute of Medicine (Committee on Quality of Health Care in America; Institute of Medicine, 2001), and is the *expected* approach to health care, implementation of LPAA values should become easier. However, as I thought about the themes in this book, the "elephant in the room,"—*funding*, loomed large. Funding will be an important consideration as we embark on the next 20 years of LPAA. Thinking outside the box will be imperative. Advocacy and awareness will be critical to directing funding to intervention that addresses meaningful outcomes. Consumer and professional organizations will need to join forces to document needs and demand services. International collaborations seeking meaningful solutions in aphasia management will help with advocacy (e.g., Collaboration of Aphasia Trialists, Aphasia United). But unless we demonstrate that our interventions make a significant difference in the daily lives of our clients, new funding streams are unlikely to materialize. Clinicians will need to implement intervention that is most effective and efficient in achieving meaningful outcomes; such approaches are not likely to include random workbook exercises or repetitious word practice. Rather, factors that lead to successfully living with aphasia, such as having friends, doing things, and feeling positive are the ultimate goals of intervention and attention to such goals must establish our treatments as necessary and effective.

As we move toward 2040, my ambition is for research and programming to routinely include LPAA values in planning and implementation. The next twenty years will be instrumental in shifting to a true partnership with people living with aphasia. This partnership will place the daily needs of people living with aphasia at the forefront. Introduction of positive psychology (Holland & Nelson, 2020) into aphasia management has encouraged us to consider possibilities, rather than listing limitations (Haley et al., 2019). With this positive orientation, I end with sincere optimism for the future. As this book demonstrates, a new generation of clinicians and researchers are leading the way!

References

Armour, M., Brady, S., Sayyad, A., & Krieger, R. (2019). Self-reported quality of life outcomes in aphasia using life participation approach values: 1-year outcomes. *Archives of Rehabilitation Research and Clinical Translation, 1*(3–4), 100025. https://doi.org/10.1016/j.arrct.2019.100025

Baar, S. (2021). Discovering functional needs in speech-language therapy. In A. Holland & R. J. Elman (Eds.), *Neurogenic communication disorders and the life participation approach: The social imperative in supporting individuals and families.* San Diego, CA: Plural Publishing.

Baier, C., Hoepner, J., & Sather, T. (2018). Exploring Snapchat as a dynamic capture tool for social networking in persons with aphasia. *Aphasiology, 32*, 1336–1359. https://doi.org/10.1080/02687038.2017.1409870

Baker, C., Worrall, L., Rose, M., Hudson, K., Ryan, B., & O'Byrne, L. (2018). A systematic review of rehabilitation interventions to prevent and treat depression in post-stroke aphasia. *Disability and Reha-*

bilitation, 40, 1870–1892. https://doi.org/10.1080/09638288.2017.1315181

Berg, K., Askim, T., Balandin, S., Armstrong, E., & Rise, M. (2017). Experiences of participation in goal setting for people with stroke-induced aphasia in Norway. A qualitative study. *Disability and Rehabilitation, 39,* 1122–1130. https://doi.org/10.1080/09638288.2016.1185167

Berg, K., Rise, M., Balandin, S., Armstrong, E., & Askim. T. (2016). Speech pathologists' experience of involving people with stroke-induced aphasia in clinical decision-making during rehabilitation. *Disability and Rehabilitation, 38,* 870–808. https://doi.org/10.3109/09638288.2015.1066453

Bernstein-Ellis, E. & Elman, R. (2006). *The Book Connection™: A life participation book club for individuals with acquired reading impairment* [Manual]. Oakland, CA: Aphasia Center of California. Retrieved from http://www.aphasiacenter.org

Brandenburg, C., Worrall, L., Copland, D., & Rodriguez, A. (2017). Barriers and facilitators to using the CommFit™ smart phone app to measure talk time for people with aphasia. *Aphasiology, 31,* 901–927. https://doi.org/10.1080/02687038.2016.1219016

Chang, H., Power, E., O'Halloran, R., & Foster, A. (2018). Stroke communication partner training: A national survey of 122 clinicians on current practice patterns and perceived implementation barriers and facilitators. *International Journal of Speech-Language Pathology, 53,* 1094–1109. https://doi.org/10.1111/1460-6984.12421

Committee on Quality of Health Care in America; Institute of Medicine. (2001). *Crossing the quality chasm: A new health system for the 21st Century.* Washington, DC: National Academy Press.

Douglas, N., & Smyth, D. (2021). Life participation for people with dementia. In A. Holland & R. J. Elman (Eds.), *Neurogenic communication disorders and the life participation approach: The social imperative in supporting individuals and families.* San Diego, CA: Plural Publishing.

Elman, R. J. (2021). C.A.P.E.: A checklist of four essential and evidence-based categories for aphasia intervention. In A. Holland & R. J. Elman (Eds.), *Neurogenic communication disorders and the life participation approach: The social imperative in supporting individuals and families.* San Diego, CA: Plural Publishing.

Epstein, R., & Street, R. (2011). The values and value of patient-centered care. *Annals of Family Medicine, 9,* 100–103. https://doi.org/10.1370/afm.1239

Grawburg, M., Howe, T., Worrall, L., & Scarinci, N. (2013) Third-party disability in family members of people with aphasia: A systematic review. *Disability and Rehabilitation, 35*(16), 1324–1341. https://doi.org/10.3109/09638288.2012.735341

Grawburg, M., Howe, T., Worrall, L., & Scarinci, N. (2014) Describing the impact of aphasia on close family members using the ICF framework. *Disability and Rehabilitation, 36*(14), 1184–1195, https://doi.org/10.3109/09638288.2013.834984

Guyatt, G., Montori, V., Devereaux, P. J., Schünemann, H., & Bhandari, M. (2004). Patients at the center: In our practice and in our use of language. *ACP Journal Club, 140,* A11–A12.

Haley, K., Cunningham, K., Barry, J., & de Riesthal, M. (2019) Collaborative goals for communicative life participation in aphasia: The FOURC model. *American Journal of Speech-Language Pathology, 28,* 1–13.

Haley, K., Womack, J., Helm-Estabrooks, N., & Lovette, B., Goff, R. (2013). Supporting autonomy for people with aphasia: Use of the Life Interests and Values (LIV) cards. *Topics in Stroke, 20*(1), 22–35. https://doi.org/10.1310/tsr2001-22

Halle, M., LeDorze, G., & Mingant, A. (2014) Speech-language therapists' process of including significant others in aphasia rehabilitation. *International Journal of Language and Communication Disorders, 49,* 748–760.

Hersh, D. (2004). Ten things our clients might say about their aphasia therapy . . . if we only asked. *ACQ Issues in Language, Speech, and Hearing, 6*(2), 102–105.

Hersh, D., Sherratt, S., Howe, T., Worrall, L., Davidson, B., & Ferguson, A. (2012). An analysis of the "goal" in aphasia rehabilitation. *Aphasiology, 26,* 971–984.

Holland, A., & Nelson, R. (2020). *Counseling in communication disorders: A wellness perspective* (3rd ed.). San Diego, CA: Plural Publishing.

Holliday, R., Antoun, M., & Playford, E. (2005). A survey of goal-setting methods used in rehabilitation. *Neurorehabilitation and Neural Repair, 19,* 227–231.

Howe, T., Davidson, B., Worrall, L., Hersh, D., Ferguson, A., Sherratt, S., & Gilbert, J. (2012). 'You needed to rehab families as well': Family members own goals for aphasia rehabilitation. *International Journal of Language and Communication Disorders, 47,* 511–521.

Kagan, A., Simmons-Mackie, N., Victor, J. C., Carling-Rowland, A., Hoch, J., Huijbregts, M., . . . Mok, A. (2011). *Assessment for Living with Aphasia (ALA).* Toronto, ON: Aphasia Institute.

Kim, E., Ruelling, A., Garcia, J., & Kainer, R. (2017). A pilot study examining the impact of aphasia camp participation on quality of life for people with aphasia. *Topics in Stroke Rehabilitation, 24,* 107–113. https://doi.org/10.1080/10749357.2016.1196907

King, J. (2013). Supporting communication with technology. In N. Simmons-Mackie, J. King, & D. Beukelman (Eds.), *Supporting communication for adults with acute and chronic aphasia* (pp. 73–98). Baltimore, MD: Brookes.

Kneebone, I. (2016). Stepped psychological care after stroke. *Disability and Rehabilitation, 38*, 1836–1843. https://doi.org/10.3109/096382 88.2015.1107764

Knollman-Porter, K., & Julian, S. (2019). Book club experiences, engagement, and reading support use by people with aphasia. *American Journal of Speech-Language Pathology, 28*, 1084–1098. https://doi .org/10.1044/2019_AJSLP-18-0237

Konnerup, U. (2017). Engaging people with aphasia in design of rehabilitation through participatory design: A way to learn what they really want. In A. Kanstrup, A. Bygholm, P. Bertelsen, & C. Nohr (Eds.), *Participatory design & health information technology.* Amsterdam, The Netherlands: IOS Press.

LPAA Project Group (Chapey, R., Duchan, J., Elman, R., Garcia, L., Kagan, A., Lyon, J., & Simmons-Mackie, N.). (2000). Life Participation Approach to Aphasia: A statement of values for the future. *ASHA Leader, 5*, 4–6.

McMenamin, R., Tierney, E., & MacFarlane, A. (2018). Using a Participatory Learning and Action (PLA) research approach to involve people with aphasia as co-researchers in service evaluation: An analysis of co-researchers' experiences. *Aphasiology, 32*(Suppl.1), 142–144. https://doi.org/10.1080/02687038.2018.1486380

Meulenbroek, P., & Keegan, L. (2021). The life participation approach and social reintegration after traumatic brain injury. In A. Holland & R. J. Elman (Eds.). *Neurogenic communication disorders and the life participation approach: The social imperative in supporting individuals and families.* San Diego, CA: Plural Publishing.

Parr, S., Byng, S., Gilpin, & S. Ireland, C. (1997). *Talking about aphasia: Living with loss of language after stroke.* Buckingham, UK: Open University Press.

Paul, N., & Sanders, G. (2010). Applying an ecological framework to education needs of communication partners of individuals with aphasia. *Aphasiology, 24*, 1095–112.

Pound, C., & Laywood, C. (2020). *Involving people with communication disability in participatory research: The friendship and aphasia project.* Retrieved from https://www.invo.org.uk/involving-people-with-communication-disability-in-participatory-research-the-friendship-and-aphasia-project/

Rohde, A., Townley-O'Neill, K., Trendall, K., Worrall, L., & Cornwell, P. (2012). A comparison of client and therapist goals for people with aphasia: A qualitative exploratory study. *Aphasiology, 26,* 1298–1315. https://doi.org/10.1080/02687038.2012.706799

Rose, M., Ferguson, A., Power, E., Togher, L., & Worrall, L. (2014). Aphasia rehabilitation in Australia: Current practices, challenges and future directions. *International Journal of Speech-Language Pathology, 16,* 169–180. https://doi.org/10.3109/17549507.2013.794474

Sather, T., & Howe, T. (2021). The role of the environment: Supporting language, communication, and participation. In A. Holland & R. J. Elman (Eds.). *Neurogenic communication disorders and the life participation approach: The social imperative in supporting individuals and families.* San Diego, CA: Plural Publishing.

Sherratt, S., Worrall, L., Pearson, C., Howe, T., Hersh, D., & Davidson, B. (2011). "Well it has to be language-related": Speech-language pathologists' goals for people with aphasia and their families. *International Journal of Speech-Language Pathology, 13,* 317–328. https://doi.org/10.3109/17549507.2011.584632

Simmons-Mackie, N. (1998). A solution to the discharge dilemma in aphasia: Social approaches to aphasia management. *Aphasiology, 12,* 231–239.

Simmons-Mackie, N. (2013). Frameworks for managing communication support for people with aphasia. In N. Simmons-Mackie, J. King, & D. Beukelman (Eds.), *Supporting communication for adults with acute and chronic aphasia* (pp. 11–50). Baltimore, MD: Brookes.

Simmons-Mackie, N. (2018). *Aphasia in North America.* Moorestown, NJ: Aphasia Access.

Simmons-Mackie, N., & Damico, J. S. (1993, November). *Towards a socially driven model of aphasic communication.* Presentation at the American Speech-Language-Hearing Association Annual Convention, Anaheim, CA.

Simmons-Mackie, N., & Damico, J. S. (1999). Social role negotiation in aphasia therapy: Competence, incompetence and conflict. In D. Kovarsky, J. Duchan, & M. Maxwell (Eds.), *Constructing (in)competence: Disabling evaluations in clinical and social interactions* (pp. 313–342). Mahwah, NJ: Erlbaum.

Simmons-Mackie, N., & Damico, J. S. (2011). Exploring clinical interaction in speech-language therapy: Narrative, discourse and relationships. In R. Fourie (Ed.), *Therapeutic processes for communication disorders* (pp. 35–52). UK: Psychology Press.

Simmons-Mackie, N., Damico, J., & Nelson, H. (1995, June). *Interactional dynamics in aphasia therapy.* Paper presented at the Clinical Aphasiology Conference, Sunriver, OR.

Srinivasan, M., Franks, P., Meredith, L., Fiscella, K., Epstein, R., & Kravitz, R. (2006). Connoisseurs of care? Unannounced standardized patients' ratings of physicians. *Medical Care, 44,* 1092–1098.

Strong, K., & Shadden, B. (2021). Stories at the heart of life participation: Both the telling and listening matter. In A. Holland & R. J. Elman (Eds.), *Neurogenic communication disorders and the life participation approach: The social imperative in supporting individuals and families*. San Diego, CA: Plural Publishing.

Sutton, M. (2020). *How to personalize impairment-based therapy: Tactus therapy tips*. (Email communication, January 29, 2020)

Szabo, G., & Dittelman, J. (2014). Using mobile technology with individuals with aphasia: Native iPad features and everyday apps. *Seminars in Speech and Language, 35*, 5–16. https://doi.org/10.1055/s-0033-1362993

Tamplin, J., Baker, F., Jones, B., Way, A., & Lee, S. (2013). 'Stroke a Chord': The effect of singing in a community choir on mood and social engagement for people living with aphasia following a stroke. *NeuroRehabilitation, 32*, 929–941. https://doi.org/10.3233/NRE-130916

The Joint Commission. (2016, February). Informed consent: More than getting a signature. *Quick Safety*. Issue 21. Retrieved from https://www.jointcommission.org/-/media/deprecated-unorganized/imported-assets/tjc/system-folders/joint-commission-online/quick_safety_issue_twenty-one_february_2016pdf.pdf?db=web&hash=5944307ED39088503A008A70D2C768AA

Torrence, J., Baylor, C., Yorkston, K., & Spencer, K. (2016). Addressing communicative participation in treatment planning for adults: A survey of U.S. speech-language pathologists. *American Journal of Speech-Language Pathology, 25*, 355–370.

Worrall, L. (2019) The seven habits of highly effective aphasia therapists: The perspective of people living with aphasia. *International Journal of Speech-Language Pathology, 21*, 438–447. https://doi.org/10.1080/17549507.2019.1660804

Worrall, L., Ryan, B., Hudson, K., Kneebone, I., Simmons-Mackie, N., Asaduzzaman, K., . . . Rose, M. (2016). Reducing the psychosocial impact of aphasia on mood and quality of life in people with aphasia and the impact of caregiving in family members through the Aphasia Action Success Knowledge (Aphasia ASK) program: A cluster randomized controlled trial. *Trials, 17*, 153.

Zumbansen, A., Peretz, I., Anglade, C., Bilodeau, J., Généreux, S., Hubert, M., & Hébert, S. (2017). Effect of choir activity in the rehabilitation of aphasia: A blind, randomised, controlled pilot study, *Aphasiology, 31*, 879–900. https://doi.org/10.1080/02687038.2016.1227424

INDEX

Note: Page numbers in **bold** reference non-text material.

Grammarly®, 151
Great Britain, 7
Group Approaches to Treatment,
6, 8–10, 12, 14–15, 26–27,
29, 33–38, 44, 55, 82, **88**,
90, 92, 94, 96–97, 115,
122–123, 139–140, **144**,
150, 153, 173, 188, 194,
198, 215
Guided Autobiography (GAB)
tool, 121
Guided models, 140

H

HARC (Houston Aphasia
Recovery Center), 12
Health, aphasia and, 107–108
Health care
patient-centered, LPAA and,
210
person centered approach, 55
Helm-Estabrooks, Nancy, 3
Hersh, Deborah, 8
Holistic framework, Life
Participation Approach to
Aphasia (LPAA), 56
Holland, Audrey, 25, 28
Hoover, Liz, 14
Houston, TX, Houston Aphasia
Recovery Center (HARC),
12
Human, interaction, stories and,
108–115

I

ICF (International Classification
of Functioning, Disability,
and Health), 28, 55
Identity, 56, 106–111, 114,
116–117, 119–125, 161,
169, 171, 175, 182–184,

186, 188–189, **190**,
196, 196, 198–199, 211,
218–219
described, 186, 188
Life Participation Approach to
Aphasia (LPAA), 218–219
stories and, 110
IFCI-SAI (*Inpatient Functional
Interview: Screening,
Assessment, and
Intervention*), 168
Illness narratives, 113–115
supporting, 120–123
Impairment
based interventions, 142
focused model, 54
*Inpatient Functional Interview:
Screening, Assessment,
and Intervention* (IFCI-
SAI), 168
Interaction, human, stories and,
108–115
Intergenerational programming,
164
International Classification of
Functioning, Disability,
and Health (ICF), World
Health Organization
(WHO), 28, 31, 55, **68**, 84
Interventions
compensatory, 142–143
functional, 139
impairment-based, 142
Life Participation Approach to
Aphasia (LPAA), 140–150
Interviewing
motivational, 59–60, **61**
examples of, **61**
TBI (Traumatic brain injury)
and, 188
person with TBI, 186–199
Isolation, TBI (Traumatic brain
injury) and, 195

J

Job Analysis Worksheet, **192**

K

Kagan, Aura, 7, 9, 11, 25
  hosts meetings, 28
Kaplan, Edith, Aphasia Grand
    Rounds and, 3

L

Laminated props, 40
Language, aphasia and, 32
*Language in Context: The
    Acquisition of Pragmatics*,
    6
Language
  interventions, primary
    progressive aphasia (PPA),
    138–140
  loss, degenerative,
    communication treatment
    in, 139
  pragmatics, 4
Lexicons, personalized, 143
*Life Interests and Values (LIV)
    Cards*, **66**, 172
Life participation
    person-centered care and,
    161–162
  stories and, 108–115
Life Participation Approach to
    Aphasia Project
  to Aphasia, 28–29
  group formed, 28
Life Participation Approach to
    Aphasia (LPAA), 10–12,
    25, 54, 55, 132
  care partners, 216–218
  choice and, 211–213
  core components of, 28–29
  discussed, 209–211

emotional experience and,
    218–219
environment, 215–216
focus on environment and,
    82
guided models, 140
holistic framework, 56
identity and, 218–219
incorporating story into,
    115–124
interventions, 140–150
outcomes, 213–215
person-centered care and,
    161–162
principles of, 11
progressive aphasia evaluation,
    136
Project group, 28
Rehabilitation Treatment
    Specification System,
    189
speech language pathologists
    and, 106
stories and, 108–115
speech language pathologists
    and, 106
traumatic brain injury and,
    182
Life Thread Model, 121
Linguistic Underpinnings of
    Narrative in Aphasia
    (LUNA), 112, 120
Listening, to stories, 106,
    116–118
  domains, 57
Living with Aphasia: Framework
    for Outcome Measurement
    (A-FROM), 12, 31, 32, 161,
    182, 186
  domains, 31, **32**
Logopenic (PPA-L), 133
Loneliness, TBI (Traumatic brain
    injury) and, 195

LPAA (Life Participation
Approach to Aphasia),
10–12, 25, 54, 132
care partners, 216–218
choice and, 211–213
core components of, 28–29
discussed, 209–211
emotional experience and,
218–219
environment, 215–216
focus on environment and, 82
guided models, 140
holistic framework, 56
identity and, 218–219
incorporating story into,
115–124
interventions, 140–150
outcomes, 213–215
principles of, 11
progressive aphasia evaluation,
136
Project group, 28
Rehabilitation Treatment
Specification System, 189
speech-language pathologists
and, 106
traumatic brain injury and,
182
LUNA (Linguistic Underpinnings
of Narrative in Aphasia),
112, 120
Lyon, Jon, 10, 11, 25
training volunteers and,
35–36

M

MacWhinney, Brian, 6
Martha's Vineyard, meetings at,
28
Maywood, NJ, 13
Adler Aphasia Center of, 12
McVicker Sally
"befriending" program, 36

Re-Connect and, 8
Mead, Margaret, 46
Measurable goals, writing,
meeting functional needs,
67–73
Meetings, client, 36–37
Memoirs, 113–115
Memory aids, external, 162–163
Mesulam, Marsel, 132
Microsoft PowerPoint®, 150
Midland, TX, 14
Model, A-FROM, 161
Modifications
environmental, 143
dementia and, 166
Montessori-based activities,
163–164
Morganstein, Shirley, "Speaking
of Aphasia," 13
Motivational interviewing, 59–60,
61
examples of, **61**
TBI (Traumatic brain injury)
and, 188
Music, dementia and, 165
"My Story" Project, 122

N

NAA (National Aphasia
Association), 5, **66**
Narrative,185, 188
illness, 113–115
supporting, 120–123
personal, 109
everyday, 112–113
identify, stories, 110
National Aphasia Association
(NAA), 5, **66**
National Center for Neurogenic
Communication Disorders,
9
National Easter Seal Society, 26
Neal, Patricia, 5–6

Physical
environmental factors, 86–89
facilitators, **87–89**
PicCollage®, 150, 151
Pinterest®, 151
Pittsburgh, PA, 8
Policy, environmental factors,
89–91
Positive Behavior Interventions
and Supports (PBIS), 195
Pound, Carole, 8
hosts meetings, 28
PowerPoint®, 150
PPA (Primary progressive
aphasia), 132–135
counseling/support, 135–136
education/counseling, 140–142
language interventions,
138–140
treatment planning, 136–137
PPAOS (Primary progressive
apraxia of speech), 134
PPA-S (Semantic), agrammatic
(PPA-G), 133
Primary progressive aphasia
(PPA), 132–135
counseling/support, 135–136
education/counseling, 140–142
language interventions,
138–140
treatment planning, 136–137
Primary progressive apraxia of
speech (PPAOS), 134
Programming, intergenerational,
164
Progressive aphasia, LPAA (Life
Participation Approach to
Aphasia) evaluation, 136
Props, laminated, 40
Prutting, Carol, 7, 24
PULSE, 119
PWA (Person with aphasia)
environments driven by, 83
voluntariness of, 92

Q

QoL (Quality of life), aphasia
and, 107–108
Quality, described, 92
Quality of life (QoL), aphasia
and, 107–108
Quest story, 113–114
Questionnaires, 39

R

Reading, physical facilitators
supporting, **87–88**
Receiving, stories, 106
Re-Connect, 8
Recovery from Aphasia, 3
Rehabilitation Institute of
Chicago, 12
Rehabilitation Treatment
Specification System, 189
Resilience, 153
Restitution story, 113–114
Restorative therapy, techniques,
106
Rich communicative
environments, 91–92
Rose, Miranda, 8
Russia, aphasia and, 2–3

S

Santa Barbara, University of
California at, 24
Santa Fe, NM, 14
Sarno, Martha Taylor, 4, 16, 28
Functional Communication
Profile and, 5–6
*Scales of Cognitive and
Communicative Ability
for Neurorehabilitation
(SCCAN)*, **69**,170,172
SCA™ (Supported Conversation
for Aphasia™), 40–42, 142

provided by Aphasia Institute, 42

SCCAN (Scales of Cognitive and Communicative Ability in Neurorehabilitation), **69**

Schuell, Hildred, aphasia and, 3

Sedona, Clinical Aphasiology Conference, 12

Semantic (PPA-S), agrammatic (PPA-G), 133

Service, environmental factors, 89–91

Setting-specific needs checklist, 62, **64**

Sexually offensive behavior, TBI (Traumatic brain injury) and, 196

S-FAVRES (Student–Functional Assessment of Verbal Reasoning and Executive Strategies), **69**

SGD (Speech-generating device), 151

Silverman, Maura, 15

Simmons-Mackie, Nina, 11, 14, 25

State of Aphasia in North America, 108

Siri®, 151

Skilled nursing facility (SNF), dementia, 169–171

SLPs (Speech-language pathologists)
Life Participation Approach to Aphasia and, 106
PPA (Primary progressive aphasia) and, 132

Small stories, 112
supporting, 120

SMARTER Goals, 67, 83, 137

Smith, Marilyn Certner, "Speaking of Aphasia," 13

SNF (Skilled nursing facility), dementia, 169–171

SNI (Social Networks Inventory), 136–137

Snyder Center for Aphasia Life Enhancement (SCALE), Baltimore, MD, 12–13

Social
cognition, TBI (Traumatic brain injury) and, 184–185
communication, TBI (Traumatic brain injury) and, 184–185
connections, integrating, 214
construction, stories and, 110
network, inventories, 39

Social Imperative, 209–210
2000–2010, 11–15
environment, five E's of, 82–83
Martha Taylor Sarno and, 5
next 50 years, 15–16
Nineties into 21st century, 9–11
Roald Dahl and, 6
seventies and eighties, 6–9
therapy and, 2

Social Imperative in Aphasia, 12

Social Imperative in the United States, history of, 9

Social Networks Inventory (SNI), 136–137

Social skills, workplace environment and, 191

South Africa, 7

Southwark, London, England, Re-Connect and, 8

Spaced retrieval training, 163

Sparks, Robert, Aphasia Grand Rounds and, 3

Spatial physical facilitators, **88**

"Speaking of Aphasia," founded, 13

"Speech Acts," 4, 7

Speech and Stroke Centre, North York, 25

Speech-generating device (SGD),
151
Speech-language pathologists
(SLPs)
Life Participation Approach to
Aphasia and, 106
PPA (Primary progressive
aphasia) and, 132
Speech-language pathology
2000-2010, 11–15
next 50 years, 15–16
Nineties into 21st century,
9–11
seventies and eighties, 6–9
Standardized assessment, case
study, 75
Standardized tests, **68–69**
*State of Aphasia in North
America*, 108
Stories
big, 113–115
supporting, 120–123
chaos, 113–114
identity and, 110
impact of aphasia, 111
incorporating into Life
Participation Approach to
Aphasia (LPAA), 115–124
life participation and, 108–115
listening to, 106, 116–118
narrative identify, 110
quest, 113–114
restitution, 113–114
small, 112
supporting, 120
social construction and, 110
support telling of, 118–120
supporting
family, 123–124
friends, 123–124
telling/listening, 106
as tools, 109
transformation through, 108
types of, 111–112

Story therapy
incorporating into Life
Participation Approach to
Aphasia (LPAA), 115–124
social imperative of
supporting, 106–108
transformation through, 108
Storytelling, 110
Strategies, communication,
148–150
Stroke Comeback Center, 12
Student training, 213
Student–Functional Assessment
of Verbal Reasoning
and Executive Strategies
(S-FAVRES), **69**
Supported Conversation for
Adults with Aphasia
(SCA™), 40–42, 142
provided by Aphasia Institute,
42
"Supported Conversation in
Aphasia," 12
*Supporting Communication for
Adults with Acute and
Chronic Aphasia*, 10
System, environmental factors,
89–91

T

Talking photo book, 39
TAP (Triangle Aphasia Project),
12
TBI (Traumatic brain injury)
communication disorders after,
181–183
emotional sequelae of, 183
Express, 198
impairments in, 183–185
cognitive-communication
difficulties, 183–184
interview/encounter,
186–199